Opening the Door to Good Nutrition

Tips for Healthy Eating, Grocery Shopping, Cooking, and Putting it All Together!

Marion J. Franz, R.D., M.S.; Betsy Kerr Hedding, R.D., M.P.H.; and Gayle Leitch, B.S.

Credits:

Editor and Production Coordinator
Michael P. Moore, B.A.
International Diabetes Center

Design and Keyline
West 44th Street Graphics
Minneapolis, Minnesota

Illustrations
Tom Foty Advertising Art
Minneapolis, Minnesota
(illus. on page 25 by Dynamic Graphics)

Printing
Associated Lithographers, Inc.
Minneapolis, Minnesota

TABLE OF CONTENTS

LIST OF TABLES

PREFACE

You may wonder why the International Diabetes Center is publishing a book on nutrition for the general public. There are several reasons. First, and probably the most important, is that the nutritional recommendations that can help everyone remain healthy are the same recommendations that are important for people with diabetes. A few specific guidelines are more important if you have diabetes, but we feel the general guidelines are equally important for all of us.

A second reason for this book is the need for sensible nutritional recommendations to deal with weight control. Obesity is strongly associated with diabetes, especially Type II or non-insulin-dependent diabetes, which is the type that people develop at an older age. If there is diabetes in your family, it is especially important for you to stay at a desirable weight. Obesity can be the lifestyle factor that brings on diabetes.

There are also other health problems that can be affected by good nutrition. These include coronary heart disease and hypertension (high blood pressure), which are major causes of death among Americans. People with diabetes are at a higher risk for developing coronary heart disease and hypertension, so it is especially important for them to make appropriate changes in their eating patterns. However, these same changes could prevent many of the deaths and much of the disability related to unhealthy eating habits among the general public.

At the International Diabetes Center in Minneapolis, we encourage the entire family to make the same nutritional changes that we recommend for the child or adult with diabetes. Not only is this a form of support for the person with diabetes, but it also benefits the entire family as well. It contributes to a healthy lifestyle for all!

Betsy, Gayle and I are involved in SHAPE, a health promotion program of the Park Nicollet Medical Foundation in Minneapolis. Betsy is a nutritionist and is Executive Director of SHAPE. Gayle is a nutritionist and a program consultant for SHAPE. All three of us have developed SHAPE's nutrition program and do much lecturing and writing in the nutrition and wellness areas.

This book is the result of our attempts to answer the question of how everyone should eat to remain healthy. More importantly, it includes the many tips we have learned and developed to help people make nutritional changes. In the process of presenting many seminars for the general public and for business executives and companies, we have often been asked *how* to successfully make changes in nutritional habits. This book contains the guidelines we use and the process everyone can follow to incorporate good nutrition into their eating habits. The ideas and suggestions that program participants have shared with us have been invaluable in helping us put together this book.

We want to thank the many individuals who have been supportive in the writing of this book: our families; the staff of the International Diabetes Center, especially Dr. Donnell Etzwiler, Bill Henry, and Mike Moore for his patience and excellent editing skills; the staff at SHAPE, especially Dr. Jim Reinertsen and Carolyn Peterson; and past SHAPE participants. Thanks to you all!

Marion J. Franz, R.D., M.S.

Director of Nutrition
International Diabetes Center
SHAPE Nutritionist

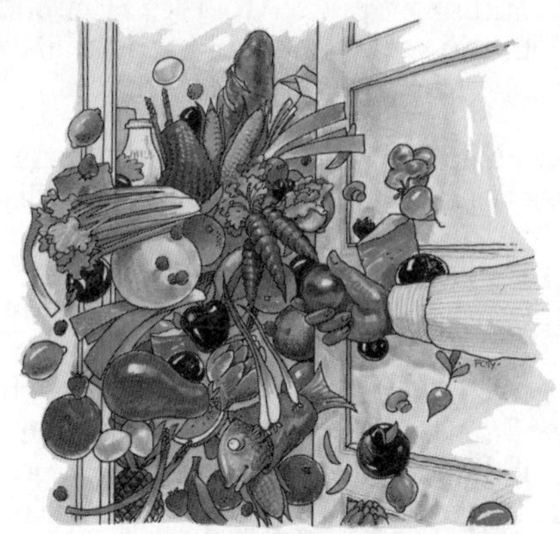

1

OPENING THE DOOR TO MAKING HEALTHY FOOD CHOICES!

Lifestyle has a strong influence on health. Statistics from the Centers for Disease Control show that 51 percent of the overall risks for the ten leading causes of death in the United States are related to lifestyle—a part of which is nutrition. The controllable lifestyle risk factors are seatbelt use; use of tobacco, alcohol, and other sedative or hypnotic drugs; mental well-being; fitness; and nutrition. You have little or no influence over the other 49 percent of the factors which contribute to your health. These include heredity, age, sex, access to medical care, and perhaps your environment. But the encouraging note is that by improving your lifestyle, you can take control of the other half!

Nutrition, one of the controllable factors, is what this book is all about. In recent years, Americans have become increasingly concerned about what we eat. A reflection of this concern is the increase in magazine articles and books about nutrition and the popularity of the so-called "health food" stores and "natural" food supplements. In fact, it has been reported that books offering diet and nutrition advice are now outselling books offering counsel about sex!

Awareness of the health benefits and risks associated with various foods has led more and more people to ask, "How should we eat to remain healthy?" With the wide variety of foods available in our society, it is a challenge to make wise food choices.

Research has shown that by controlling certain dietary substances you can reduce your risks of developing coronary heart disease (blockage of the blood vessels in and near the heart), hypertension (high blood pressure), stroke (blockage of blood vessels to the brain), obesity, non-insulin-dependent diabetes (which usually occurs in adults), dental caries (cavities), cirrhosis (fibrous blockage) of the liver, and some forms of cancer (breast, colon, prostate, stomach and esophagus). If any of these diseases run in your family, you should be particularly careful of the risk factors and do what you can to prevent these diseases from happening to you. As an example, if diabetes is common in your family, you should do what you can to prevent obesity, which is a strong risk factor for diabetes.

Nutrition changes start with the family. Such changes are important for children and youths as well as adults. Research has shown that many of our eating habits are learned at a young age, and health problems that are related to poor diet often start developing when a person is young. This was shown with distressing clarity when autopsies of American soldiers killed in the Korean War revealed that 42 percent had arteries clogged and hardened by deposits of cholesterol, which is a sign of a disease called atherosclerosis, a process which can lead to coronary heart disease. The average age of these men was only 22! In contrast, the arteries of Japanese natives the same age, who had been raised on a diet of rice and vegetables, showed no such damage in autopsies.

In the past 100 years, the eating patterns of Americans have changed drastically—and most of the changes have NOT been to our benefit. For example:

- In 1981, the average man, woman, and child in the United States consumed approximately 125 pounds of fat. About 40 to 50 percent of our total caloric intake is fat, which is about 20 percent more than Americans ate 60 years ago, and nearly three times the amount consumed by the Japanese and some African and Latin American populations. The Human Nutrition Information Service (HNIS) of the United States Department of Agriculture (USDA) reported that in 1982, 34 percent of the fat in the average American diet came from meat, poultry and fish; 12 percent from dairy products; 44 percent from fats and oils; and the rest from a variety of food products.

- Today, the average American consumes approximately 100 to 130 pounds of sugar a year. That's the equivalent of 600 calories per person each day! This includes all sugars, of which an average of 71 pounds is from sucrose—table sugar. Most of the remaining sugar is from corn syrups. Of the approximately 60 pounds of corn syrups used, high fructose corn syrup (HFCS) accounts for 38 pounds, and its commercial use is increasing. Refined sugars and other nutritive sweeteners (syrups, corn syrup, honey, molasses) supply 18 to 25 percent of the average American's total energy intake. Sugar is the leading food additive in the United States. It has been suggested that sugar should contribute no more than 10 percent of total energy intake. Although there is no current evidence to indicate health hazards from sugar (except cavities), it can provide excess calories and therefore contribute to obesity.

- The soft drink industry is the largest purchaser of sugar. Consumption of soft drinks has doubled since 1962, and they have become the most popular beverage for Americans. In 1962 coffee was the leading beverage purchased, followed by milk, alcoholic beverages, soft drinks, and tea and fruit juices. But by 1982 soft drinks rose to nearly 30 percent of the market, while alcoholic beverages—of which beer is the main component—increased their share to 21 percent, in second place. Milk dropped to third place with 20 percent consumption; coffee to fourth place, 18 percent of the market; and tea and fruit juices remained in last place with 10 percent. In 1981, an average American drank 412 twelve-ounce servings of soda pop, which was a 25 percent increase from 1976! Soft drinks account for about one-fourth of our total sugar intake, or 23 pounds of sugar per person per year.

- After sugar, salt is the next leading food additive. The average American consumes 10 to 20 grams, or about 2 to 4 teaspoons of salt each day, which is about 20 times the needed amount and two to four times the recommended amount. This adds up to 15 pounds of salt per person per year.

- In the early 1900s, 40 percent of our calories came from fruits, vegetables, and grain products. That figure is now only 20 percent, with 60 percent of our calories coming from fats and refined and processed sugars.

- Overeating is a major health problem. Almost 30 percent of men age 30 to 60 and 20 percent of women age 30 to 60 are above desirable body weight, while total daily caloric intake per person has dropped about 3 percent since 1910. Americans are now more sedentary, so less is still far too much.

The above dietary changes have had a major impact on our health. Over-consumption of foods high in calories and fat (especially saturated fat and cholesterol), refined and processed sugars, salt, and alcohol has been associated with the development of a number of disorders. These include heart disease, some cancers, hypertension, stroke, diabetes, and cirrhosis of the liver.

Diet As a Risk Factor in Heart Disease

Research has shown a connection between diet and cardiovascular disease (disease of the heart and its blood vessels). In a landmark seven-nation study conducted in 1947 by Ancel Keys, a direct correlation was discovered between a country's incidence of heart disease, the level of cholesterol in its people, and the amount and type of fat in the national diet. The Finns, with the diet highest in dairy fat, had the highest average cholesterol level (250-300 mg/dl) and the highest rate of heart disease. People in the United States, with a diet also high in total fat, were close behind, with an average cholesterol level of 200-250 mg/dl. But the Japanese, who eat a diet low in total fat and dairy fat, had the lowest average cholesterol level (140-160 mg/dl) and the least amount of cardiovascular disease. Their rate of fatal heart attacks was one fourth the United States rate. Another study showed that when Japanese emigrated to the United States and adopted a Western diet, their incidence of fatal heart attacks climbed to ten times that of their countrymen in Japan.

However, even though numerous studies over the ensuing years pointed to the fact that lowering the level of cholesterol in the blood was beneficial, doubt still remained in some scientists' minds. Each of the studies had design flaws or possible contributing factors other than diet, so researchers were reluctant to conclude that reducing the level of blood cholesterol would reduce the risk of heart disease.

Then in January 1984, the results were announced of an elaborate, ten-year study conducted by the National Heart, Lung, and Blood Institute (NHLBI). According to Columbia University cardiologist Robert Levy, who directed the study, there no longer is any doubt that lowering cholesterol levels lowers the risk of heart disease and saves lives.

The NHLBI study had recruited 3,086 men between the ages of 35 and 59, all of whom had cholesterol levels above 265 mg/dl. Half of the men were put on daily doses of cholestyramine, a cholesterol-lowering drug, and the other half received a similar looking and tasting placebo (inactive substance). It was decided to use a drug rather than diet to lower cholesterol because it would have been virtually impossible to control or measure the diet of so many men over so long a period.

By the end of the study, the cholestyramine group had achieved an average cholesterol level 11 percent lower than that of the control

group and had suffered 19 percent fewer heart attacks. Their cardiac death rate was a remarkable 24 percent lower than that of the placebo group. This meant that for every 1 percent reduction in total cholesterol level, there was more than a 2 percent reduction in incidence of heart disease. Furthermore, men who lowered their cholesterol level the most—a 35 percent reduction—had a 49 percent reduction in occurrence of fatal and non-fatal heart attacks.
Can this reduction in risk of heart disease be achieved just by improving the diet? And if so would this benefit all Americans? According to Levy, "If we can get everyone to lower cholesterol 10 to 15 percent by cutting down on fat and cholesterol in the diet, heart-attack deaths in this country will decrease by 20 to 30 percent. A reasonable goal for most individuals would be a cholesterol level under 200 mg/dl.

The next step was to resolve some of the questions about the link between blood cholesterol levels and heart disease, and to define steps that should be taken to diagnose and treat elevated blood cholesterol levels. In December 1984, the NHLBI and the National Institutes of Health (NIH) convened a Consensus Development Conference on Lowering Blood Cholesterol to Prevent Heart Disease. The result was a recommendation that diet be used as the first means to achieve the goal of reducing the blood cholesterol level of the entire adult population to less than 200 mg/dl, and to less than 180 mg/dl in those under age 30. Furthermore, it was emphasized that all Americans (except children under the age of 2) need to adopt a diet that reduces fat and cholesterol intake.

Atherosclerosis (clogging and hardening of the arteries, which can lead to coronary heart disease) is believed to begin when the lining of an artery is damaged. Damage can be caused by high blood pressure, chemicals from cigarette smoke, or elevated levels of blood fats (cholesterol). Smoking, high blood pressure and elevated cholesterol also appear to interfere with the normal arterial healing process. As a result, platelets, connective tissue, and large white blood cells called "macrophages" accumulate in the damaged artery walls.

The macrophages fill up with cholesterol from the blood, forming a "foam cell." When they burst, a fatty deposit called "plaque" begins. This plaque may cease to develop or even shrink in size when cholesterol levels are reduced. More often, however, the continued insults of rich foods, and smoking will lead over a period of time to a gradual increase in the size of the plaque. Coronary heart disease is produced by cholesterol-laden blood constantly flowing over the damaged and plaque-lined walls of the arteries. Finally, the flow of blood may become obstructed. If this happens in an artery in or near the heart, chest pain results. If the artery is completely blocked, a heart attack occurs. If the blocked artery is one that delivers blood to the brain, the outcome will be a stroke. Often there are no warning signs of the existence or progression of coronary heart disease. For up to one third of the victims, the first sign of the disease is the heart attack which causes sudden death.

Cholesterol and similar fatty substances (collectively referred to as lipids) must be transported through the bloodstream. Since they are unable to dissolve in the blood, the body packages them with proteins in envelopes called "lipoproteins." Lipoproteins can be divided into three major families:

Very low density lipoproteins (VLDL), which carry fat (triglycerides) in the blood and a small amount of cholesterol.

Low density lipoproteins (LDL), which carry the majority of the cholesterol in the blood. LDL scoops up cholesterol absorbed from digesting food in the intestines and the cholesterol made in the liver and carries it throughout the body.

High density lipoproteins (HDL), which carry the rest of the cholesterol.

LDL cholesterol can be thought of as potentially on its way to the artery wall, where it can become part of the fatty plaque. The HDL cholesterol, on the other hand, is thought to be on its way back to the liver, where it will be removed from the body. Too much LDL and not enough HDL may lead to a situation in which cholesterol builds up in the artery wall, causing atherosclerosis and coronary heart disease. Diets high in fat, particularly saturated fats, cause the LDL cholesterol in the blood to increase. People who exercise regularly have been shown to have higher levels of HDL cholesterol than do sedentary persons.

One of the major factors in the prevention of coronary heart disease is to eat a diet that reduces the amount of cholesterol in the blood. Specifically, it is recommended that the total amount of fat in the diet be reduced by decreasing consumption of saturated fats and cholesterol, which are generally found in animal foods. Saturated fats interfere with the way the body handles cholesterol. The amount of fiber in the diet also seems to influence cholesterol levels. When foods high in fiber are eaten, the fiber seems to interfere with absorption. This results in less cholesterol being absorbed from the small intestine into the bloodstream. Types of fiber that are especially helpful in reducing cholesterol are found in legumes (beans, peas, lentils), fruit, and oat bran.

The American Heart Association recommends the following dietary strategy:

1. Adjust caloric intake to achieve and maintain ideal body

weight. Obesity frequently occurs along with high blood pressure, diabetes, and elevated blood cholesterol levels. All are high risk factors for coronary heart disease.

2. Reduce the total amount of calories from fat from the current average of 40% to about 30-35%. Saturated fats should account for less than 10% of the total calories while polyunsaturated fats should supply up to 10%. (Types of fat in foods will be discussed in later chapters.)

3. Substantially reduce dietary cholesterol. The average daily intake of cholesterol by adults should be less than 300 milligrams.

4. Increase amount of total calories coming from carbohydrate foods, especially complex carbohydrates (starches and fiber).

5. Avoid excessive amounts of sodium in the diet, because a high sodium intake has been associated with high blood pressure, which is a well-recognized risk factor in coronary heart disease.

6. If alcohol is consumed, do so only in moderation (a maximum of 2-3 drinks a day for nonpregnant adults). Alcohol can contribute a significant amount of calories to the diet.

Diet As a Risk Factor in Cancer

"Eat all your vegetables, Hilary, a new study shows that eating lots of vegetables reduces the risk of cancer," reports Sally Forth to her daughter Hilary in the June 28, 1984 comic strip by Greg Howard. And Hilary replies, "Why is it always something like vegetables? Why couldn't it have been chocolate chip cookies?"

The relationship of eating habits to cancer prevention is an area of research that recently has been generating a great deal of interest. The available evidence recently led three eminent organizations, the American Cancer Society; the Committee on Diet, Nutrition, and Cancer of the National Academy of Sciences; and the U.S. Department of Health and Human Services, to band together and issue guidelines urging Americans to adopt eating habits associated with reduced risk of cancer. The Committee of the National Academy of Sciences compared the current state of knowledge about the effect diet has on cancer to the knowledge that existed 20 years ago about cigarettes and lung cancer. Although there is mounting evidence, little of it is considered to be as conclusive as the cigarette/lung cancer evidence now is. However, the committee decided there was enough evidence to support interim guidelines on diet and cancer.

The American Cancer Society in 1984 issued the following recommendations suggesting how nutrition may reduce cancer risk.

1. ***Avoid obesity.*** Studies have found increased rates of cancer of the uterus, kidneys, stomach, colon and breast in people who are 40 percent or more overweight.

2. ***Cut down on fat intake in order to lower the risk of breast, colon and prostate cancer.*** The consumption of both saturated fats and unsaturated fats should be reduced in the U.S. diet from the existing average of 40 percent to about 30 percent. Studies show that the amount of fat in the diet can affect the levels of hormones (in particular, prolactin, estrogen and androgens) which are linked to the development of cancer of the breast and prostate. In colon cancer, studies suggest that high levels of dietary fat cause increased secretion of bile acids into the intestinal tract. Several bile acids have been shown to cause cancer in animals.

3. ***Eat more high fiber foods, such as fruits, vegetables and whole grain cereals.***The increased fiber from fruits and vegetables and whole grain cereals and breads speeds the passage of other foods through the intestine, which may reduce the chance for cancer-causing chemicals to have an effect.

4. ***Include foods rich in vitamins A and C in the daily diet.*** Especially important are citrus fruits, which are high in vitamin C, and dark green and deep yellow vegetables, which are high in beta carotene that the body converts into vitamin A. Studies have shown that these two vitamins may help prevent some forms of cancer. But the committee strongly warned against supplementing the diet with pill forms of these vitamins, since high doses can have serious side effects. You can get all the vitamins A and C your body can use by choosing two helpings daily from the fruit and vegetables mentioned above.

5. ***Include cruciferous vegetables such as cabbage, broccoli, Brussels sprouts, kohlrabi and cauliflower in the diet.*** Evidence from laboratory experiments suggests that some non-nutritive chemicals present in cruciferous vegetables may inhibit the formation of cancer-causing chemicals or reduce cancer incidence in other ways.

6. ***If you drink alcohol, do not drink excessively.*** Excessive alcohol consumption has been linked to an increase in incidence of colon and rectal cancer. The combination of

excessive drinking and smoking seems to increase the risk of cancer of the mouth, larynx, esophagus and respiratory tract.

7. ***Be moderate in consumption of salt-cured, smoked and nitrite-cured foods.*** Studies of populations in some parts of the world that frequently consume these foods have shown that they have a greater incidence of some cancers, particularly cancer of the stomach and esophagus. Some methods of smoking and pickling foods seem to produce greater amounts of hydrocarbons and nitrosamines, which have been shown to cause cancer in laboratory animals.

The American Cancer Society report also reviewed other diet-cancer questions, but because of insufficient evidence made no recommendations for warnings against food additives, saccharin or other artificial sweeteners, coffee or caffeine, fried or broiled foods, or dietary cholesterol. The American Cancer Society also felt there wasn't enough evidence to support cancer-prevention values of other vitamins or selenium. What is known about the above substances follows:

Food additives. Knowledge about the possible cancer risks or benefits of food additives is insufficient to warrant a recommendation for or against their use. Those additives which have been found to cause cancer are already banned.

Vitamin E. There is no evidence that vitamin E prevents cancer in humans, although antioxidants such as vitamin E have been shown to prevent some cancer in animal research.

Selenium. Evidence that selenium protects against some cancers is limited, and because of the danger of selenium poisoning, warnings have been issued against medically unsupervised use of selenium as a food supplement.

Artificial sweeteners. There is no evidence that moderate use of saccharin or other non-caloric sweeteners causes cancer in humans.

Coffee. Although studies of populations of heavy coffee drinkers have shown weak links between heavy coffee drinking and bladder and pancreas cancers, there is no evidence that caffeine causes cancer in humans.

Meat and fish cooked at high temperatures, such as frying or broiling. Recent studies have demonstrated that high temperature frying or broiling creates substances (mutagens) which can induce cancer in animals, and the subject is being studied further.

Cholesterol. Evidence relating both high and low blood cholesterol levels to human cancers is inconclusive.

The National Cancer Institute's recommendations for preventing cancer ("Cancer Prevention Awareness Program") includes the following seven guidelines:

1. Don't smoke or use tobacco in any form.
2. Make changes in your diet to increase your intake of fiber and reduce the fat you eat.
3. If you drink alcoholic beverages, do so only in moderation—one or two drinks a day.
4. In the workplace, know and follow the rules for health and safety.
5. Avoid x-rays unless they are medically necessary.
6. Protect your skin from overexposure to sunlight.
7. Take estrogens only as long as necessary.

As you can see, the recommendations to reduce the risk of cancer are healthy and sensible changes. In fact, they are similar to the nutritional guidelines to reduce the risk of coronary heart disease.

Diet As a Risk Factor in Hypertension

Hypertension (high blood pressure) is a serious health problem today in the United States. About 18 percent of the population—some 60 million Americans—suffer from this disorder. About 90 percent of these cases of hypertension are medically classified as "essential," which means the cause is unknown. Whether or not the cause is known, attempts should be made to control hypertension as soon as it is discovered. Uncontrolled hypertension is hazardous to health in many ways. It is the leading cause of stroke and contributes to heart and kidney disease.

Blood pressure is always reported in two figures: first a larger number and then a smaller number. The larger number is called the systolic pressure, and it is the amount of pressure exerted on the walls of the blood vessels (arteries) when the heart is at the strongest point in its contractions (beats). The smaller number, called the diastolic pressure, is the amount of pressure left in the arteries when the heart is resting between contractions. It is desirable for adults to have a blood pressure reading of 120/80 or lower. Consistent readings greater than 140/90 require a doctor's attention.

Although the exact cause of an individual's hypertension is often unknown, various factors are thought to be potential culprits in raising blood pressure:

Genetics. Heredity has a strong influence on an individual's blood pressure. It seems that there must be a genetic susceptibility before an individual can develop hypertension. The problem is that most people do not know what their genes "have in store" for them.

Salt. Sodium, a major component of table salt, is thought to be the main dietary culprit in hypertension. Populations with a high average daily intake of sodium have been shown to have a high rate of hypertension. Some individuals seem to inherit a problem in which their kidneys have a reduced ability to remove sodium from the body, and this increases their chances of developing hypertension. For these reasons, sodium moderation is important in preventing hypertension, and sodium restriction is an important aspect of management of existing hypertension.

Excess salt consumption creates a situation in the fluid surrounding the body's cells in which extra fluid must be retained to balance the extra sodium. This extra fluid surrounding the cells results in increased pressure on the arteries. The excess fluids also increase the volume of the blood circulating in the body. This requires the heart to exert a greater force to pump the extra fluid through the blood vessels, thus increasing blood pressure.

Obesity. There is a close association between obesity and hypertension. Weight loss decreases blood pressure substantially, and often even a loss of 5 to 10 pounds can make a big difference.

Tobacco smoking. Smoking causes a narrowing or tightening of the blood vessels, which causes the heart to work harder to pump blood through them.

High fat, high cholesterol diet. If the arteries become clogged with plaque buildup and fatty deposits, the heart again must work harder to pump blood through them, and the pressure inside the arteries increases as they become more and more clogged. This process can result in hypertension and may be an early sign of coronary heart disease.

Stress. Stressful moments in life can temporarily raise blood pressure, but stress itself does not necessarily lead to hypertension. However, a large amount of psychological stress over many years may contribute to hypertension.

Calcium. Recent studies have suggested that problems with the body's use of calcium may also be involved in causing hypertension. A diet containing adequate amounts of calcium has been shown to lower blood pressure.

Potassium. Other studies have pointed to a dietary deficiency of potassium as a factor in the development of hypertension.

Alcohol. People who have a high alcohol intake also tend to have high blood pressure.

The National High Blood Pressure Program of the National Heart, Lung, and Blood Institute recommends the following six changes in diet and lifestyle to reduce high blood pressure:

1. Weight reduction should be the first step for people who are more than 20 pounds over their desirable weight or have a high percentage of body fat. Weight reduction by caloric restriction often results in a substantial lowering of blood pressure.

2. A reduced sodium diet is recommended for people with a family history of hypertension, which is the only "genetic marker" currently known. Studies have proven again and again that a diet high in salt has a detrimental effect on blood pressure and that reducing salt intake can help to lower it. Restricting daily sodium intake to approximately 2 grams of sodium (2300 milligrams) or 5 grams of salt may reduce elevated blood pressure. Reducing sodium may also reduce the loss of potassium that often results from diuretic therapy (use of pills to remove excess body fluid and ease pressure on blood vessels).

3. Those who drink should do so in moderation, consuming not more than 2 ounces of alcohol per day (2 ounces of 100 proof liquor, 8 ounces of wine, or 24 ounces of beer).

4. Reduce intake of foods containing saturated fats, replacing them with unsaturated fats and complex carbohydrates.

5. Do not smoke.

6. Regular exercise is encouraged, and has been found effective in lowering blood pressure whether or not the exerciser is obese.

Reducing blood pressure decreases cardiovascular problems in individuals with moderate to severe hypertension. For those with mild hypertension who are at low risk of heart disease, lifestyle changes as listed above should be pursued aggressively while blood pressure is carefully monitored.

Evidence associating potassium, calcium, and magnesium with hypertension is less convincing than for the above changes. However, the following suggestions have been made:

- High intake of potassium-rich foods can help ease hypertension and can also protect against its onset. Foods high in potassium and low in sodium and calories include low-fat milk, bananas, apricots, grapefruit, oranges, tomatoes, broccoli, Brussels sprouts, carrots, cauliflower, mushrooms, winter squash, sweet and white potatoes, corn and spinach.

- Increasing intake of calcium-rich foods has been shown in some studies to help protect against hypertension and aid in its treatment, but this is still controversial. The best sources of calcium are low-fat milk products.

- Increasing intake of magnesium-rich foods helps maintain regular heartbeat and assists in the contraction and relaxation of muscles and arteries. The best sources of magnesium are almonds, beans, bran, brown rice, hazel nuts, lentils, oats, peanuts, and whole-wheat and whole-rye flour.

As you can see, a number of factors can cause blood pressure to creep upward, leading to potentially serious problems. A generally healthy diet can help prevent high blood pressure, and specific nutritional and lifestyle changes mentioned can keep it from advancing to a damaging stage if it already exists.

Diet As a Risk Factor in Diabetes

There are two types of diabetes. Insulin-dependent (Type I) diabetes occurs suddenly, usually in children or young adults; it can occur in older lean adults, but it is more common in young individuals. In this type of diabetes, the pancreas stops producing insulin, a hormone the body needs to properly convert food to energy. As a result, the person becomes very thin, tired, and sometimes very sick. These people then need to take daily insulin shots and follow individualized meal and exercise plans to help their bodies use food for energy and growth. Diet is not a factor in causing Type I diabetes, but it is important in controlling it once it occurs. Because these people must inject insulin to stay alive, Type I diabetes is also known as "insulin-dependent" diabetes.

Non-insulin-dependent (Type II) diabetes occurs in adults, often progressing gradually without causing any symptoms. It occurs when the body's insulin is no longer effective enough to keep the amount of glucose (sugar from digested food) in the blood at a normal level. The blood glucose level remains consistently elevated in these people until they are diagnosed by a blood or urine test and begin treatment of Type II diabetes. Diet is a major factor in causing Type II diabetes, because 80 to 90 percent of the people who develop it are obese. Obesity can cause the body to become resistant to the action of its own insulin. The pancreas of these people is often producing more than the normal amount of insulin, but the body's cells are resistant to the insulin and therefore blood glucose levels become elevated.

Diet is also a major factor in controlling Type II diabetes, because a combination of an individualized meal plan and regular exercise program will often keep the person's blood glucose within normal range. If the person is obese, weight loss will often help control Type II diabetes. Sometimes a diabetes pill (oral hypoglycemic agent) or insulin must be used to help control Type II diabetes, but the person is not dependent on the medication in the sense that the person with Type I diabetes needs insulin to stay alive. This is why Type II diabetes is referred to as non-insulin-dependent diabetes.

It is important to maintain good control of the blood glucose and blood lipid (fat) levels in both Type I and II diabetes. Consistently high levels can, over the years, cause serious problems such as heart, eye and kidney disease, nerve damage and blood circulation problems.

It is not yet known how to prevent Type I diabetes, but there are strong indications that Type II diabetes can be prevented by good nutrition and maintaining a normal body weight. For individuals who have a family history of Type II diabetes, it is especially important to make lifestyle changes, if necessary, to prevent the development of the disease. Blood glucose levels should be checked annually, especially after reaching the age of 30.

Persons who already have Type II diabetes may be able to improve their health by making positive changes in lifestyle, with emphasis on good nutrition and regular exercise. These changes will help to minimize the impact diabetes has on their lives.

The American Diabetes Association has made the following general nutritional recommendations:

1. Weight reduction is the primary objective of therapy for most people with Type II diabetes, because they are usually obese.

2. Dietary sources of saturated fats and cholesterol should be restricted. About 75 percent of the deaths among people with diabetes can be attributed to atherosclerosis.

3. Natural sources of unrefined carbohydrates and fiber should be substituted for foods which contain refined sugar and no or little fiber.

4. Avoid nutritionally unbalanced "fad" diets.

5. Consider moderate restriction of salt intake.

6. There is not enough evidence to either encourage or discourage the use of alternative sweeteners such as saccharin, aspartame, fructose, xylitol, sorbitol and mannitol.

7. If approved by an individual's physician, a moderate amount of alcohol may be consumed.

Diet As a Risk Factor in Cirrhosis of the Liver

Cirrhosis of the liver is a condition in which there is excessive formation of connective tissue in the liver, causing blockage that decreases the liver's ability to help in the metabolism (use) of foods. Excessive alcohol consumption is the primary factor in causing cirrhosis of the liver, which is the ninth leading killer disease of Americans.

The liver is the organ most involved in breaking down alcohol after it is consumed. Alcohol is both a toxic substance (poison) and a source of calories. The body must use valuable nutrients to detoxify alcohol that is consumed. An ounce of an alcoholic beverage contains about 80 to 90 calories, but no vitamins or minerals. In other words, alcohol can contribute to a calorie surplus in the diet, while actually reducing the nutritional value of the total food intake.

The average American of drinking age consumes about 210 calories of alcohol per day. The total volume of distilled alcohol, wine and beer consumed in the United States every year breaks down to an average of 2.6 gallons per person; however, alcohol consumption varies among individuals probably more than does any other category in the diet.

Not only is alcohol a factor in cirrhosis of the liver, it is also a very dangerous substance if used by pregnant women. Alcohol crosses the placenta to the fetus and can damage the health and development of the baby. Since no one knows at the present time if there is a "safe" level of alcohol intake during pregnancy, it is best for pregnant women to abstain from drinking altogether. The liver can metabolize about an ounce of alcohol per hour. Amounts above this level leave the liver and enter the general bloodstream. Circulating blood then reaches the placenta, and alcohol can cross the placenta to the fetus. The fetus then literally becomes drunk. Excessive alcohol is especially damaging to the fetus early in pregnancy. Problems may include slowing of growth and development and damage to mental development which may result in a lowering of intelligence quotient (IQ).

Diet As a Risk Factor in Osteoporosis

Although not among the ten leading causes of death in the United States, osteoporosis is another serious health problem that is affected by nutrition. Osteoporosis is a condition in which the bones become fragile, causing even minor collisions or falls to result in painful and disabling fractures, principally of the spine, hip and wrist. An estimated 15 million people in the United States have osteoporosis, including one of every four women over the age of 60. Approximately 90 percent of all fractures in people over age 60 are related to osteoporosis, and it is the underlying cause of many of the 190,000 hip fractures reported annually.

Research has started to shed some light on possible causes of osteoporosis. Four factors seem to be involved:

1. ***Heredity,*** however, genetics is still beyond our control.
2. ***Poor nutrition,*** especially a dietary deficiency of calcium.
3. ***Hormones,*** especially the decreased amount of estrogen produced by the ovaries after menopause.
4. ***Lack of exercise,*** or general lack of stress on the bones as a result of inactivity.

Nutrition

Children ages one to ten and nonpregnant adults need a minimum of 800 to 1,200 milligrams of calcium per day. Teenagers, pregnant women and possibly the elderly need a minimum of 1,200 to 1,500 milligrams of calcium per day. Because of the high incidence of osteoporosis in American women, some researchers recommend that women also have a daily intake of 1,200 to 1,500 milligrams of calcium. Most women however, are reluctant to consume the number of calories needed to ingest more than 1,000 milligrams of calcium each day. Calcium carbonate (powdered egg shells) is a good calcium supplement to the diets of these women. Another supplement that might be considered is the stomach acid neutralizer "Tums"; one Tums tablet contains 200 milligrams of calcium. For increased absorption, calcium supplements should be taken between meals and preferably with milk or yogurt. Avoid bone meal or dolomite as a calcium supplement, because both have a high lead content, which is toxic to the body.

Besides calcium intake, other dietary factors affect the way calcium is absorbed by the bones. Vitamin D is needed for the proper absorption of calcium and to assist the movement of calcium from the blood to the bones. However, few people are at risk of a vitamin D deficiency if they have even minimal exposure to the sun. Fifteen minutes per day exposure to sun is adequate for vitamin D synthesis. Large amounts of protein and fiber can decrease calcium absorption. Lactose, the carbohydrate found in milk, enhances calcium absorption.

Exercise
Substantial evidence now shows that exercise increases bone strength. Regularly exercised bones respond to the extra stress by increasing their calcium deposits, which makes the bones stronger. For all the bones of the body to benefit from this strengthening, you must follow a complete exercise program that stresses all parts of the body.

Hormones
Recent evidence has encouraged physicians to prescribe estrogen for women who have lower levels of natural estrogen after menopause. Many physicians believe that this estrogen therapy is safe, and if used in an appropriate manner, its benefits outweigh any risks.

Sources of Calcium
All dairy products are good sources of calcium. Three fourths of Americans' dietary calcium comes from milk, yogurt, cheese, ice cream and other dairy products. In order to keep the percentage of calories from fat and total calories in the recommended ranges, calcium sources should be from products that are low in saturated fat and cholesterol. Choose the skim or low-fat products of milk, cheese, cottage cheese, and yogurt; and eat ice milk instead of ice cream. Sardines and salmon with bones, oysters (packed in water and rinsed to remove salt), broccoli and other "greens," and tofu can be other low-fat calcium sources.

The table on the next page lists common food sources of calcium:

CALCIUM CONTENT OF DAIRY PRODUCTS AND OTHER COMMON FOODS

Food	Serving Size	Calcium (milligrams)
Yogurt (plain, lowfat)	1 cup	350-450
Dry, lowfat milk	¼ cup	
Sardines with bones	3 oz.	
Fruit-flavored yogurt	1 cup	250-350
All milks	1 cup	
Swiss cheese	1 oz.	
Buttermilk	1 cup	
Hard cheese	1 oz.	150-250
Processed cheese	1 oz.	
Salmon with bones	3 oz.	
Oysters	1 cup (10-11 medium)	
Tofu	4 oz.	
Soft cheeses	1 oz.	50-150
Cooked dried beans	1 cup	
Ice cream or ice milk	½ cup	
Cottage cheese	½ cup	
Almonds	1 oz.	
Broccoli	½ cup	
Orange	1	
Spinach, cooked	½ cup	
Kale, cooked	½ cup	

WHICH SUPPLEMENT IS BEST?

Calcium supplements*

Listed by types; within types, listed in order of increasing cost.

Product (manufacturer)	Calcium per tablet (milligrams)
Calcium carbonate tablets	
TUMS ANTACID (Norcliff-Thayer)	200
CALTRATE 600 (Lederle)	600
BIOCAL (Miles)	500
CALCIUM CARBONATE (Lilly)	260
ALKA-2 CHEWABLE ANTACID (Miles)	200
OS-CAL (Marion)	500
BIOCAL (Miles)	250
Calcium lactate tablets	
CALCIUM LACTATE (General Nutrition Corp.)	100
NATURAL CALCIUM LACTATE (Schiff)	100
FORMULA 81 (Plus)	83
CALCIUM LACTATE (Lilly)	84
Calcium gluconate tablets	
CALCIUM GLUCONATE (Pioneer)	62
CALCIUM GLUCONATE (Lilly)	47
Chelated calcium tablets**	
CHELATED CALCIUM (Solgar)	167
CALCIUM OROTATE 2000 (Nature's Plus)	100
CALCIUM OROTATE (KAL)	50

* Adapted from **Consumer Reports** October 1984.

** Chelation anchors the calcium to other chemicals, which supposedly improves absorption in the intestine. But according to **Consumer Reports** (October 1984) chelation does nothing but raise the price of the tablets.

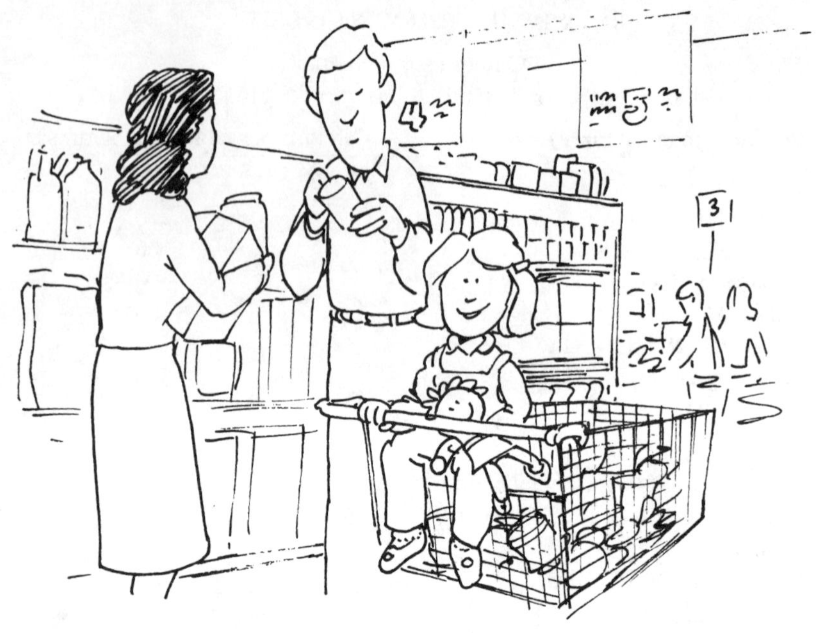

Getting Started

You can open the door to nutrition by making the following basic guidelines part of your lifestyle. This eating pattern assures that you will meet the nutritional recommendations we have discussed with each of the diseases that have diet as a risk factor.

The philosopher Kant once said, "It is often necessary to make a decision on the basis of knowledge sufficient for action but insufficient to satisfy the intellect." Sushma Palmer of the National Academy of Sciences in Washington, D.C., points out that controversy about dietary guidelines is usually philosophical. Two schools of thought emerge about how scientific evidence should be applied to the development of public nutritional recommendations. One school asserts that a complete understanding of how and why a benefit occurs as well as absolute proof of the benefit is necessary before offering advice to the general population. The other school contends that recommendations for the general population should be made when various pieces of evidence suggest that eating habits are associated with risk of chronic disease. The proposed dietary recommendations should provide a high likelihood of benefit with a minimal chance of harm.

The chart on page 26 summarizes the various nutritional recommendations by government, voluntary, and public health agencies. As you see, there is a remarkable amount of agreement among a wide variety of groups about dietary recommendations.

Achievement of desirable body weight to avoid obesity is uniformly recommended. Generally an increase in complex carbohydrate with emphasis on dietary fiber, and a decrease in simple sugar is also suggested. A reduction in sodium intake to reduce risk of hypertension is also generally recommended. Despite a great deal of difference in the philosophy for decision making and unresolved differences on some specific recommendations, it is amazing how similar the nutrition advice is by these different groups!

However, remember that changes in eating habits are no "guarantee" that a disease will not happen to you. They are important for general good health. The best advice is still to avoid obesity, don't smoke, if you drink alcohol do so in moderation, eat a varied and well-balanced diet, and exercise regularly.

These guidelines are the basis for the explanations and tips in the rest of the book:

- **Maintain ideal weight.**
- **Eat a variety of foods.**
- **Eat plenty of fruits, vegetables and whole grains.**
- **Limit the amount of fat you eat, especially saturated fats and cholesterol.**
- **Limit the amount of salt you use.**
- **Limit the amount of sugar and sweets you eat.**
- **Limit alcohol intake to moderate amounts or avoid entirely.**

A healthy basic eating pattern, from which you can develop your personal eating plan based on your tastes and caloric needs, is shown below:

RECOMMENDED DAILY EATING PATTERN*

1. Low-fat breads, cereals, grains, rice, and pastas.	Four or more servings.
2. Fruits and vegetables.	Four or more.
3. Non-fat and low-fat dairy products.	Two or more servings.
4. Fish, poultry, lean meats, cheeses.	Six ounces or less.
5. Beans, peas, lentils, nuts, seeds.	As often as possible in place of meat.

* Use this basic pattern to develop a personal eating plan which includes your food tastes and caloric needs and meets your nutritional goals.

A Word About Changing Your Eating Habits . . . .

As you gradually change your eating habits, remember the old adage: "Variety is the spice of life." Everyone needs about 40 different nutrients to stay healthy. And since no single food supplies all the nutrients needed for an adequate diet, a variety of foods is a must. The greater the variety, the less likely you are to develop either a deficiency or an excess of any single nutrient. Another bonus of eating a variety of foods is that it reduces the chance of eating a significant amount of any food additive or contaminant that may be harmful. This may provide some reassurance in these times of increased concern about food-raising practices and mechanically mass-produced food products.

As you think about healthy eating, keep in mind that your goals are: good food, good health AND good taste. Too often we equate a diet rich in fats, cholesterol, sugar, calories and salt with good-tasting food. We assume that any sacrifice of these ingredients will automatically reduce the taste and enjoyment we get from our food. The problem is that many of us have become used to craving excessive amounts of these ingredients, and we often close our minds to healthier and equally enjoyable food choices.

The sad truth is that three out of every five calories Americans eat come from either fat and/or sugar and at least 20 percent of adults are obese. These factors are killing thousands of us every year and limiting the lifestyles of millions more. The happy truth is that with gradual and moderate changes in our eating habits, we can live much better and probably longer, and look better as well!! This book can help you take a big step in that direction. With apologies to Neil Armstrong, the first man on the moon, "This will be a giant step for an individual, and a small step for Mankind."

You are what you eat.
What will you be today?

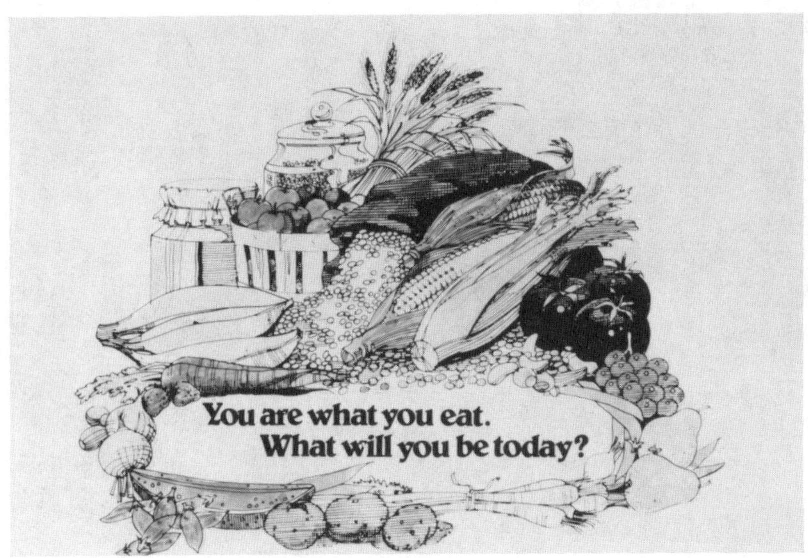

SUMMARY OF NUTRITIONAL RECOMMENDATIONS

Categories	Dietary Guidelines for Americans (1985)	Amer. Heart Assoc. (1984)	Amer. Cancer Society (1984)	Amer. Diabetes Assoc. (1979)	Blood Pressure Education Program: (1984) [NHBLI]
Calories/Body Weight	Maintain reasonable weight.	Caloric intake adjusted to achieve and maintain ideal body weight.	Avoid obesity.	Appropriate calorie control. Weight reduction in Type II diabetes.	Weight reduction, if more than 20 pounds over desirable weight.
Total Fat	Avoid too much fat.	Reduce fat to 30-35% of total calories.	Reduce from current average of 40% to about 30% of total.	Lower to 30-35%.	No recommendation.
Type of Fat	Limit saturated fat.	Less than 10% saturated. Up to 10% polyunsaturated.	Reduce both saturated and unsaturated fats.	Restrict saturated fat.	Reduce saturated fat; put more emphasis on unsaturated.
Cholesterol	Limit foods with cholesterol.	Reduce to less than 300 mg./day.	No recommendation.	Restrict foods with cholesterol.	Reduce when feasible.
Total Carbohydrate	Eat foods with adequate starch.	Make up calories lost from fat by eating carbohydrates.	No recommendation.	Raise to 45-60% of total energy value of diet.	No recommendation.
Fiber	Add fiber.	No recommendation.	Eat more high fiber foods — fruits, vegetables, whole-grain cereals.	Substitute natural unrefined CHO foods with fiber for refined CHO foods.	No recommendation.
Sugar	Avoid too much sugar.	No recommendation.	No recommendation.	Limit to modest amount.	No recommendation.
Sodium	Avoid too much sodium.	Avoid excessive sodium in diet.	Be modest in amount of salt-cured, smoked, and nitrite-cured foods.	Use moderation in salt intake.	Moderate sodium restriction — 2 grams sodium or 5 grams salt.
Alcohol	If you drink, do so in moderation—and don't drive.	Be aware of large amounts of calories that can add to diet.	Do not drink excessively.	Alcoholic beverages may be used in prescribed amounts.	Limit to moderate intake — 2 oz. per day.
Other	Eat a variety of foods.	Role of fiber, coffee, trace minerals, hardness of water, vitamins all under review.	Include foods rich in Vitamins A and C. Include cruciferous vegetables.	Avoid nutritionally unbalanced "fad diets".	Get regular aerobic exercise. Specific recommendations not made for increasing potassium, calcium, and magnesium.

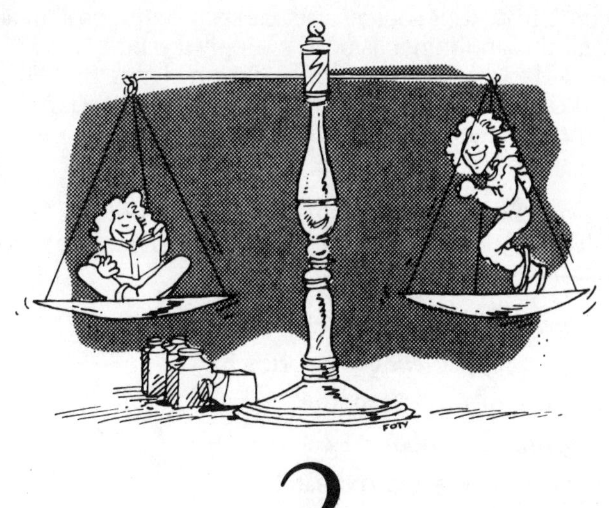

2

NUTRITIONAL KEY NUMBER ONE: LIGHTEN UP!

To "Open the Door to Nutrition" and a healthier lifestyle, the first "key" is to adjust your caloric intake and activity patterns to achieve and maintain a reasonable body weight. It can be dangerous to be overweight. Obesity is associated with Type II diabetes, high blood pressure, and increased levels of blood fats (cholesterol and triglycerides), as well as many other health problems.

Calories that are consumed in excess of your body's needs are stored as energy reserves—which is a nice way of saying fat! (Americans aren't fat, we just have plenty of energy reserves!) Fat is a very efficient means of storage, and the body has an almost limitless capacity to accumulate fatty tissue. The fact that many Americans are overnourished suggests that a vast majority of individuals are in positive energy balance—they consume more energy than they expend and stash away the surplus in fat deposits.

To lose weight, you must burn more calories than you take in. You can do this temporarily by selecting foods containing fewer calories, but to maintain desirable weight you must also make permanent changes in your eating habits and activity level. To ensure permanent success, you must be willing to commit yourself to some form of regular exercise program to change your activity level. And if you need to lose weight, do so gradually—one to two pounds per week.

Calories come from four sources: fats, carbohydrates, protein and alcohol. Vitamins and minerals do not supply the body with calories but are needed to release energy from carbohydrates, protein and fat for use by the body. Vitamins and minerals are also used to maintain the body's normal function and to keep various body processes functioning smoothly.

Most foods contain calories from more than one source. The following list outlines the number of calories supplied by various nutrients:

One gram of carbohydrate = 4 calories

One gram of protein = 4 calories

One gram of fat = 9 calories

One gram of alcohol = 7 calories

(One ounce = approximately 28 grams)

As you can see, ounce per ounce, fat has twice as many calories as protein or carbohydrate.

The typical American diet contains:

30 to 40 percent of calories from carbohydrate

15 to 18 percent of calories from protein

40 to 50 percent of calories from fat

Health professionals have recommended that Americans shift to the following percentages for a more healthy eating style:

50 to 60 percent of calories from carbohydrate

15 to 18 percent of calories from protein

25 to 30 percent of calories from fat (not more than 35 percent)

Determining Your Desirable Body Weight

The two terms often used interchangeably to describe excess body weight are "obesity" and "overweight," but they do not necessarily mean the same thing. Obesity is an excessive amount of fat regardless of actual weight in pounds. Overweight is excessive heaviness which may or may not include an excessive amount of fat. Overweight may simply mean more lean body tissue, such as muscle. Excessive fat is our main concern. People who do very little exercise may weigh an appropriate amount for their height, but they still can be obese, because too large a percentage of their weight may be from fat. On the other hand, athletes may weigh more than a height and weight table would suggest they should, but because much of their weight is from muscle, we would not classify them as being obese.

It would be ideal if we could use the actual percentage of fat on a person's body to help that person decide on an appropriate body weight. This percentage of fat can be closely estimated by a trained professional. American adult women have an average of 22 to 25 percent body fat. More than 30 percent is considered obesity. An ideal amount is 20 to 21 percent. Men average 17 to 19 percent body fat. More than 25 percent is considered obesity, and an ideal amount is 13 to 17 percent.

However, since professional help to determine your percent body fat may not be available, you can use the following steps to help you do the next best thing. This will help you find an approximate desirable body weight (DBW) and your approximate need for calories:

Women: 100 pounds for the first 5 feet
5 pounds for each additional inch
Your DBW is:________

Men: 106 pounds for the first 5 feet
6 pounds for each additional inch
Your DBW is:________

(Add 10% for large body frame; subtract 10% for small body frame.)

If you are unsure of your frame size, the following table may help. You can measure your wrist with a tape measure to determine if you are small, medium or large boned. This will give you an approximate guide.

WRIST MEASUREMENT

Height	Small Boned	Medium Boned	Large Boned
For Women:			
Under 5′2″	Less than 5½″	5½″ to 5¾″	Over 5¾″
5′2″ to 5′5″	Less than 6″	6″ to 6¼″	Over 6¼″
Over 5′5″	Less than 6¼″	6¼″ to 6½″	Over 6½″
For Men:			
Over 5′5″	5½″ to 6½″	6½″ to 7½″	Over 7½″

To maintain weight, you need approximately the following number of calories per day:

18 calories per pound of DBW if very physically active.

15 calories per pound of DBW for normal activity and if desirable body weight.

13 calories per pound of DBW after age 55 or for light activity level.

10 calories per pound of DBW if very obese or sedentary.

Your Daily Caloric Requirement: ______________________

To lose one pound of fat in a week, you need to consume 3,500 calories less than your weekly requirements, because one pound of body fat contains approximately 3,500 calories! The most effective way to use up that many calories is to reduce your caloric intake and increase your caloric expenditure. If you eat 500 calories less, you will create an energy deficit of 500 calories per day, and you will lose approximately one pound per week. If you exercise to burn 250 calories more each day, you create an additional energy deficit of one-half pound per week. To lose two pounds per week, you must create a deficit of 1,000 calories from your daily caloric requirement.

Your Daily Caloric Requirement: ______________________

minus

Daily Caloric Intake for Weight Loss: ______________________

equals

Total Caloric Intake for Weight Loss: ______________________

The lowest daily caloric intake recommended for women is 1,200 calories; 1,500 calories is the daily minimum for men. To lose more weight, increase your caloric expenditure through exercise.

Keys to Permanent Weight Control:

1. ***Modify food intake*** (eat less fat and other high calorie foods, divide food intake throughout the entire day).

2. ***Increase energy expenditure*** (exercise).

3. ***Change food-related habits*** (behavior modification techniques).

Modify Food Intake

Use the following table to determine the approximate calories in a serving of food:

APPROXIMATE CALORIC CONTENT OF FOODS		
Food Groups	**Examples of Portions**	**Calories**
1. Dairy Products	1 glass skim milk or 1 oz. skim milk cheese	80
2. Vegetables	½ cup cooked ¾ to 1 cup raw	25
3. Fruits	1 small fresh ½ cup canned without sugar	40
4. Starches	1 slice bread, ½ to ¾ cup cereal, 1 small potato, ½ cup pasta or rice, 1 muffin, etc.	70
5. Meat	1 oz. chicken, fish, ham, or lean beef, cooked	55
	1 oz. beef or pork, cooked; 1 egg; 1 oz. skim milk cheese	80
6. Fat	1 Tbsp. salad dressing, 1 tsp. margarine	45

The following are examples of 1,200 and 1,500 calorie meal plans that follow the Recommended Daily Eating Pattern:

1,200 CALORIE WEIGHT-LOSS MEAL PLAN

Food Groups	Calories		Sample Menu
Breakfast:			
1 fruit	40		½ grapefruit
1 starch	70		½ cup cooked oatmeal
½ milk	40		½ cup skim milk
		150	
Lunch:			
1 fruit	40		1 small apple
0-1 vegetable	20		carrot sticks
			Sandwich
2 starch	140		2 slices whole wheat bread
2 lean meat	110		2 oz. sliced turkey breast
1 fat	45		1 tsp. margarine
1 milk	80		1 cup skim milk
		435	
Dinner:			
1 fruit	40		¼ cantaloupe
2 vegetables	50		½ cup cooked green beans, tossed salad, lettuce with other raw vegetables
1 starch	70		1 small baked potato
3 med. fat meats	240		3 oz. roast beef
2 fats	90		1 Tbsp. salad dressing 1 tsp. margarine
½ milk	40		½ cup skim milk
		530	
Snack:			
1 starch	70		3 cups popcorn
		70	
	1,185 calories		

1,500 CALORIE WEIGHT-LOSS MEAL PLAN

Food Group	Calories		Sample Menu
Breakfast:			
1 fruit	40		½ banana
2 starches	140		1 English muffin
½ milk	40		½ cup skim milk
		220	
Lunch:			
1 fruit	40		1 small orange
0-1 vegetable	20		carrot and celery sticks
			Sandwich
2 starches	140		2 slices whole wheat bread
2 lean meats	110		2 oz. water packed tuna
1 fat	45		1 tsp. mayonnaise
1 milk	80		1 cup skim milk
		435	
Dinner:			
1 fruit	40		10-12 grapes
2 vegetables	50		½ cup cooked broccoli, tossed dinner salad with raw vegetables
4 med. fat meat	320		4 oz. broiled ground beef patty
2 starches	140		1 whole wheat roll ½ cup brown rice
3 fats	135		1 Tbsp. salad dressing 2 tsp. margarine
½ milk	40		½ cup skim milk
		725	
Snacks:			
1 starch	70		3 cups popcorn
1 fruit	40		1 small apple
		110	
		1,490 calories	

"I never eat breakfast or lunch, why am I fat?" This is a common complaint from persons struggling with weight control. What happens to the majority of these persons, if they are honest about the amount of foods eaten, is that they consume as much, if not more calories later in the day as do persons who eat regular meals at more appropriate times. Their appetite gets out of control and they become "binge eaters."

"But I'm not hungry at breakfast or lunch so why should I eat?" is the next question asked. In order to control appetite, individuals need to learn to eat at appropriate times and not wait so long that once they begin to eat they can no longer control how much they eat. Research has shown that our bodies can handle the calories eaten in smaller amounts throughout the day better than if all the calories are consumed in one large meal later in the day. And of course, if 2,500 calories have been eaten during an evening, the person won't be hungry at breakfast! Individuals need to learn to divide these calories into smaller amounts spread throughout the entire day.

"Weight control is something of which you are able—just cut down the amount of food on your table."

Increase Energy Expenditure

Exercise is an important part of a healthy lifestyle, because besides being fun, it helps to burn calories, regulate appetite, change body composition, increase basal metabolic rate (calories used at rest), and replace stress eating.

THINK ABOUT THIS! One hour, deep thought, sitting down = 90 calories. One hour, deep thought, jogging = 600 calories.

BURNING UP THOSE CALORIES!*

Activity	Time Needed To Use 250 Calories	Calories Used Per Hour of Activity
Rest and Light Activity (50-200 calories per hour)		
Lying down or sleeping	3 hrs., 8 min.	80
Sitting	2 hrs., 30 min.	100
Driving an automobile	2 hrs.	120
Fishing	1 hr., 50 min.	130
Standing	1 hr., 45 min.	140
Domestic work	1 hr., 23 min.	180

continued

Moderate Activity (200-350 calories per hour)		
Bowling	1 hr., 15 min.	200
Bicycling (5½ mph)	1 hr., 10 min.	210
Walking (2½ mph)**	1 hr., 10 min.	210
Gardening	1 hr., 8 min.	220
Canoeing (2½ mph)	1 hr., 4 min.	230
Yoga	1 hr., 4 min.	230
Golf	1 hr.	250
Lawn mowing (power mower)	1 hr.	250
Lawn mowing (hand mower)	55 min.	270
Rowboating (2½ mph)	50 min.	300
Swimming	50 min.	300
Hiking (20 lb. pack, 2 mph)	50 min.	300
Walking (3¾ mph)	50 min.	300
Dancing (slow step)	50 min.	300
Tennis (doubles, recreational)	50 min.	300
Softball	45 min.	325
Badminton	40 min.	350
Horseback riding (trotting)	40 min.	350
Square dancing	40 min.	350
Volleyball	40 min.	350
Rollerskating	40 min.	350
Vigorous Activity (over 350 calories per hour)		
Mini-trampoline	38 min.	400
Ditch digging (hand shovel)	38 min.	400
Shoveling	38 min.	400
Ice skating (10 mph)	38 min.	400
Wood chopping or sawing	38 min.	400
Bicycling (10 mph)	36 min.	415
Tennis, singles	35 min.	420
Dancing (aerobic)	33 min.	445
Hiking (20 lb. pack, 4 mph)	31 min.	450
Waterskiing	32 min.	460
Dancing (fast step)	30 min.	490
Jogging	26 min.	585
Skiing (downhill)	25 min.	600
Squash	25 min.	600
Soccer	25 min.	600
Rope skipping (90-100 skips/minute)	23 min.	655

continued

Bicycling (13 mph)	22 min.	660
Dancing, aerobic (very vigorous)	22 min.	660
Running (8 1/2 mph)	21 min.	700
Handball (2 people)	20 min.	775
Singles racquetball	20 min.	775
Skiing (cross-country)	15 min.	900

*Approximate energy expenditure by a 150-pound person in various activities. Adapted from *The Athlete's Kitchen* by Nancy Clark and from Health and Fitness News Service.

**Walking or jogging = 100 calories per mile — cover 2.5 miles for 250 calories.

Your own basal metabolic rate (BMR) will account for much of your caloric expenditure. Your BMR is based on involuntary activities such as digestion, respiration, heartbeat, and brain function as well as your age, sex, size and physical activity level. Metabolic rates decrease with age and increase with amount of muscle tissue. Since lean tissue burns more calories than does fat, a physically fit person with a low percentage of body fat will require more calories than will a person with a high percentage of body fat, even when their weights are the same.

Physical activity can also significantly increase BMR—and not just during exercise. Once your metabolic rate is increased it takes many hours to return to normal. In this way, regular aerobic exercise results in a metabolism that burns more calories—even while you sleep!

Physical activity also aids in weight loss by reducing your appetite. During and after exercise, your thirst increases but desire for food decreases. It is important to drink plenty of water to replace body fluid lost during exercise. But the decreased hunger should help you meet your caloric reduction goal. Exercise also prevents loss of muscle tissue during dieting, whereas a significantly reduced caloric intake without exercise can result in 25 to 50 percent of the weight loss being muscle.

Furthermore, if you attempt to lose weight by just dieting and not exercising, your body will adapt to the lesser amount of calories and use them more efficiently. It can lower its basal metabolic rate to help prevent starvation. So eventually cutting back on calories reaches the point of no return. The alternative is to become involved in a regular aerobic exercise program to increase your metabolic rate and burn up additional calories.

Change Food-Related Habits

To make changes in your eating habits, you must become aware of certain behaviors that go along with food selection and eating habits.

There is a difference between hunger and appetite. Hunger is your body's need for food, and appetite is your mind's desire for food. Ideally, we should use hunger as the "signal" to eat but many individuals are signaled to eat by sights, thoughts, activities, people, etc. If you discover that you are a person who eats in response to environmental signals, there are several techniques you can use to control these signals.

1. Slow down your eating speed. You'll be less likely to finish off a second helping before your body has had a chance to tell you it was satisfied with the first. Some helpful hints to reduce your eating pace are:

    - Try to take 30 minutes for meals and 15 minutes for snacks.
    - Put down your utensil between bites. Do not put it back into food until you have swallowed what is in your mouth.
    - Count your chews per bite. Take 15 chews per bite.
    - When 3/4 of the meal is finished, stop eating for five minutes. At the end of this time, if you feel like eating more, continue. If you don't feel like eating, stop and congratulate yourself.
    - If you want to take second helpings, wait ten minutes before serving yourself seconds.

2. Always eat in one location and set a full place setting for any food or beverage you take. This will reduce the number of locations you associate with food and make it difficult to "eat on the run." Other strategies for mealtime are:

    - Use a small plate for your meal rather than a full dinner plate. This will make it seem like you are getting more food.
    - Do not serve food family-style. Instead, leave all foods on the stove or in the refrigerator and serve from there.
    - Get someone else in the family to clear the plates and put away leftovers. This reduces the chance to nibble after you have finished your meal.

3. Concentrate on eating. Take in the sight, smell, texture, and taste of your food. Not only will this help slow your eating speed, but it will also make any meal more satisfying. As you concentrate, you will begin to identify unconscious eating behaviors you need to eliminate.

4. Store food out of sight and out of reach. Some of the following strategies may be helpful.

   - Do not leave any food on the counter or table in plain view—this tests your willpower too much.
   - Rearrange your cupboards and your refrigerator to reduce the exposure of tempting foods.
   - Try to spend less time in the kitchen where you are surrounded by food.
   - Avoid buying foods you tend to overeat, especially high calorie foods. They will be out of reach if you have to walk to the grocery store rather than the kitchen to find them.

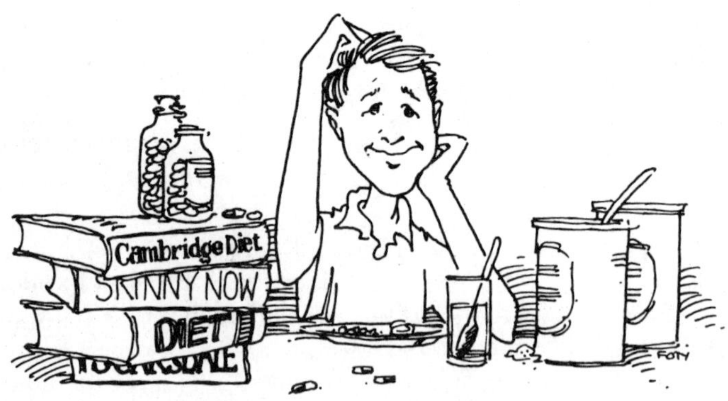

Why Fad Diets Don't Work

Any diet that promises that you can lose five to ten pounds in a week is not being realistic. As you can see from the table of caloric requirements and the amount of calories stored in fat, this is physiologically impossible. (Example: Jogging burns 100 calories a mile, so to burn the 35,000 calories in ten pounds of fat, you would have to run 350 miles!)

What happens is that most fad diets are extremely low in carbohydrates or calories. Whenever you cut back severely in carbohydrates or calories you will have a rapid loss of body fluid, which will result in a loss of weight on the scale. Unfortunately, it isn't fat you have lost, only fluid. Your body doesn't like to be dehydrated and your thirst mechanism will take over, quickly restoring those pounds of lost fluid. To gain back a pound of fluid you only have to drink one pint of liquid. You then have the "yo-yo" method of weight reduction. A realistic expectation is to lose one to two pounds per week of body fat.

New and supposedly miraculous ways of losing weight are almost daily brought to the attention of the consuming public. Why are these various weight reduction methods so appealing? Because most of them appear to promise a way to lose weight effortlessly and in a short time. Some of the characteristics of popular "fad" diets are:

Temporary: a new fad diet seems to appear every week.

Irrational: Most fad diets distort or ignore principles of good nutrition. There may be over-emphasis on one food or food group, assigning almost magical powers to it.

Something for nothing: Beware of the "calories don't count" type of diet.

Limited variety: Fad diets provide limited choices and are difficult to sustain.

In addition fad diets are:

Expensive!

Nutritionally unbalanced and can be medically dangerous.

Likely to cause loss of lean body tissue and body fluids with little loss of body fat.

Unfortunately, there is no quick and easy formula for long-lasting weight management. The secret of permanent weight management lies in establishing healthy patterns of eating and activity for a lifetime. Remember, if any of the diet schemes worked, we wouldn't need a new fad diet or diet book every month. We would have solved the problem!

Recommendations for Weight Management

For weight loss to be successful, you must remember the following guidelines:

1. Consume 500 to 1,000 calories less than your usual daily intake.
2. Participate in aerobic activities to increase muscle tissue and burn more calories.
3. Make permanent changes in eating behaviors.
4. Maintain a gradual weight loss of one to two pounds per week, until you reach your desirable weight.

It is essential to make proper eating habits and regular physical activity a permanent part of your lifestyle in order to maintain desirable body weight.

Successful permanent weight loss is a lifetime decision!

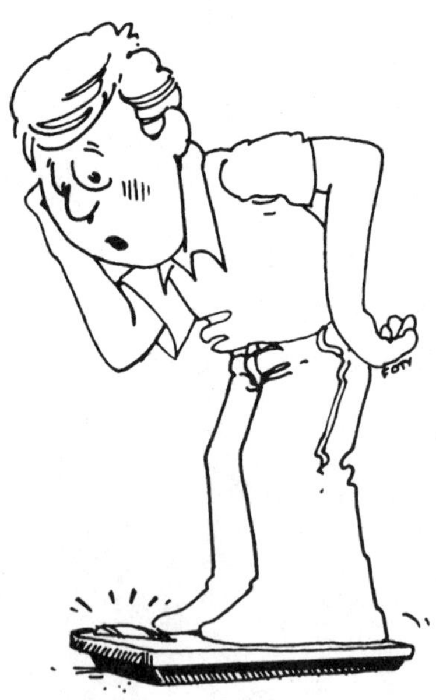

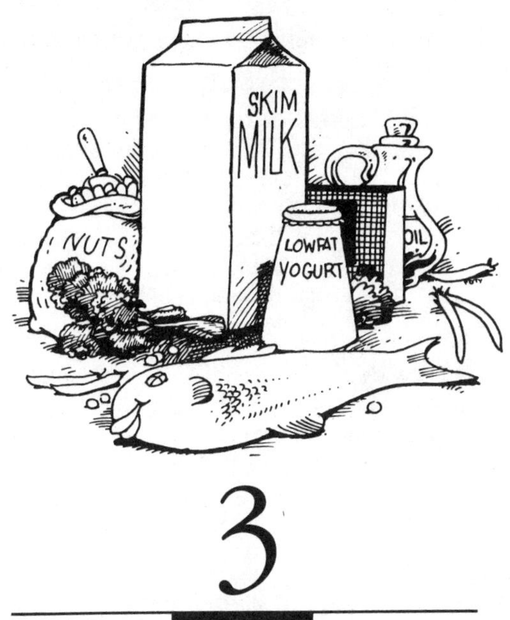

3

TRIM FAT! LEAN TOWARD LEAN!

The second key to opening the door to good nutrition and a healthy lifestyle is to limit total fat in the diet to no more than 30 to 35 percent of the daily calories and to restrict saturated fat. Saturated fat has the effect of raising blood cholesterol levels and thus increasing the risk of heart disease. It is found in animal products, coconut and palm oil used in many commercial food products, cocoa butter (chocolate), solid shortenings, and dairy products that contain butterfat. It is solid at room temperature. Whenever possible, use polyunsaturated fats in place of saturated fats. The polyunsaturated fats are found in vegetable oils such as corn, cottonseed, safflower, sunflower, sesame and soybean oils; in fish; and in some margarines. Polyunsaturated fats tend to lower blood cholesterol levels. They are liquid at room temperature.

Of course, fats cannot be totally avoided. They have important functions in our diet: transport of fat-soluble vitamins A, D, E, K; adding flavor to foods; and giving a feeling of fullness. But fats are also a highly concentrated source of energy (calories). Consequently, foods high in fat are also high in calories.

Fats can also contribute to obesity. The average American diet contains 40 to 50 percent of the calories as fat. Because of the caloric density of fat, we need to watch fat intake in order to maintain or attain ideal body weight.

Fats can be from either animal or vegetable foods, and there are different types of fat in the diet. We have defined saturated and polyunsaturated fats, but there are also monounsaturated fats. They provide fat-dense calories, but recent research indicates they may help lower blood cholesterol levels. Examples are olives and olive oil, peanuts, peanut butter and peanut oil, avocados, nuts (except the walnut, which is polyunsaturated), and seafood.

Fats differ in other important ways. Some fat is visible in food, but a large proportion is hidden, or "invisible" fat. By referring to food nutrient breakdown charts, you can find the average amount and type of fat in various foods. Watch for the term "hydrogenated" on ingredient labels. Hydrogenation is a chemical process whereby a liquid oil is hardened to make a solid fat. During the process the oil becomes saturated. Try to avoid products that contain hydrogenated or "hardened" fats.

Triglycerides are another type of fat and one of the forms in which fat is carried in the blood. Triglycerides are manufactured by our bodies from excess calories. Fats that we do not use as an energy source are also stored as triglycerides.

As discussed in the section on diet and coronary heart disease, fats are transported throughout the body as lipoproteins (a combination of fat and protein). Diets high in saturated fat seem to cause high blood levels of low density lipoprotein (LDL). LDL picks up the cholesterol globules absorbed from the intestinal tract or that are manufactured in the liver and carries them throughout the body. Very low density lipoprotein (VLDL) carries triglycerides in the blood and distributes them to fat cells for storage. Most experts agree that lowering LDL cholesterol by decreasing saturated fat intake is important in reducing the risk of coronary heart disease.

Another type of lipoprotein is the high density lipoprotein (HDL), which appears to protect against heart disease. HDL carries cholesterol from the body's tissues back to the liver where it can be excreted in bile. The amount of HDL in the blood is not as closely related to how we eat as it is to how much we exercise; people who exercise regularly have high levels of HDL.

Cholesterol is a fat-like waxy substance required by the body in small amounts. It is used by the body as building blocks for the cells and to produce certain hormones. Cholesterol in the blood comes partly from our bodies, which manufacture it in sufficient quantities to meet our needs, and partly from the foods we eat, especially fats. Dietary cholesterol is found only in animal products, especially egg yolk and organ meats such as liver. Therefore, our food choices can influence our blood cholesterol levels.

High blood cholesterol levels, which are associated with coronary heart disease, occur in populations consuming diets high in calories, total fat and saturated fats. People who have diabetes have a high risk of developing heart disease and therefore must be especially careful of fat intake.

The amount of dietary cholesterol recommended is controversial. The typical American consumes 450 to 800 milligrams of cholesterol in food each day. The American Heart Association recommends limiting it to 300 milligrams. As a rule, foods high in fat are also high in cholesterol. By reducing total fat, the amount of cholesterol will also be reduced. The following table lists foods containing cholesterol and the milligrams of cholesterol per serving size:

CHOLESTEROL SOURCES

Food	Amount	Cholesterol (milligrams)
Liver	3 oz.	372
Eggs	1 large	252
Shellfish (shrimp)	3 oz.	128*
Frankfurter	2 (4 oz.)	112
Veal, lamb, beef	3 oz.	80-86
Poultry (chicken)	3 oz.	74
Fish	3 oz.	43-60
Butter	1 Tbsp.	35
Dairy products (whole milk)	1 cup	34
Ice cream	½ cup	27-49
American cheese	1 oz.	28
Cottage cheese	½ cup	12-24
Yogurt	1 cup	17
Skim milk	1 cup	5
Desserts and baked products	avg. serving	20-150

Note: Plant sources, such as peanut butter, bread, margarines, shortenings, grains, fruits and vegetables do not contain cholesterol. Cholesterol is only found in animal fats.

*New analyses report shellfish, including shrimp, cholesterol values at 60 to 120 milligrams per three ounces.

From: U.S. Department of Agriculture, Agriculture Handbook No. 456, 1975.

The recommendation to reduce fat, especially saturated fat, can be achieved in the following ways:

- Lower total meat consumption. Limit meat, fish, poultry, cheese and eggs to six ounces or less daily (two small servings). An example to illustrate what happens to fat and calorie content as protein sizes decrease:

Meat Portions	Fat (grams)	Calories
Broiled tenderloin, 12 oz.	26.0	700
Broiled tenderloin, 8 oz.	17.5	470
Broiled tenderloin, 4 oz.	6.5	175

- Select the leanest cuts and remove all visible fat before cooking and eating.
- Increase use of vegetable protein (legumes, beans, peas, nuts and seeds) in place of animal protein.
- Use poultry (preferably without skin), fish and vegetarian meals to replace red meat whenever possible.
- Avoid high fat meats such as luncheon meats, frankfurters, sausage and bacon.
- Decrease total fat intake by baking, broiling, roasting, grilling or boiling foods. Avoid frying. Skim fat from broths, soups and gravies.
- Drink skim milk.
- Use low-fat or nonfat dairy products, such as plain yogurt and part skim milk cheese. Avoid dairy products containing large amounts of butterfat.
- Use margarine instead of butter. Be sure a liquid oil is listed as the first ingredient on the margarine label.
- Avoid food products having the term "hardened" or "hydrogenated" vegetable oil as a major ingredient.
- Use vegetable oils in your baking, cooking and salad dressings.
- Select fresh fruit, fruit-based and low-fat dairy products for dessert. Decrease intake of rich desserts.

- Be more aware of hidden fat in foods such as hamburgers, ice cream, french fries, baked products, whole milk, potato chips and many other processed foods.

The following table illustrates the difference in fat and caloric content when hamburger is compared to chicken and fish, and when pie is compared to fresh fruits:

Food Choices	**Fat (grams)**	**Calories**
Broiled hamburger, 4 oz.	13.0	250
Broiled cod, 4 oz.	6.0	187
Broiled chicken, 4 oz.	4.0	188
Pecan pie, 1/6 pie	31.6	577
Banana custard pie, 1/6 pie	14.8	353
Fresh fruit pie, 1/6 pie	17.5	404
Fresh fruit, 1 average portion	0	60

Because fat is so high in calories, the key to cutting back on fat and calories is to adapt cooking methods and recipes, reducing or eliminating butter, margarine, oil, mayonnaise, lard and salad dressing. In adapting favorite recipes, start by experimenting with cutting fat by a third or a half. This can be done most easily in casseroles and baked products and by substituting low fat cooking methods.

When recipes require sauteing in oil or butter, cut the amount in half, or better yet, use water or broth; or in place of sauteing, soften the food ingredient in a microwave oven. In cutting back on fat you may lose some moisture and flavor, so make up the difference with broth, skim milk, wine or fruit juice.

Food groups which are the major contributors of fat to the American diet are:

- *Meat, fish, poultry*
- *Dairy products*
- *Fats and oils*

Meat, Fish and Poultry

Meat is a good source of protein, iron and B vitamins. But it is also high in saturated fat, cholesterol and calories. To reduce fat intake, begin by selecting the leaner cuts of meat. Leaner meat actually contains slightly more protein, vitamins and minerals per pound than expensive fattier grades of meat. Animals accumulate fat as they age, so veal and lamb are lower in fat than meat from older animals. Grain feeding also produces greater fat content, so grass-fed beef has less marbling and fat covering.

Protein usually coexists with fat. The person who eats large portions of high-protein foods such as steaks, chops, hamburgers and cheese, is actually eating large amounts of fat. The fat calories in these foods exceed the protein calories. Most marbled meats contain 80 percent fat calories and 20 percent protein calories.

The total amount of red meat eaten by Americans in a year, as measured by retail weight, generally increased from the 1930s until 1976, when it reached its highest level of 94.4 pounds per person. From there it has dropped significantly. From 1979 to 1983, the U.S. Department of Agriculture reports it has remained between 76.5 and 78.8 pounds per person each year.

The following tables list the fat and caloric content of some average portions of meat and deli products. To reduce fat in your diet, you must remember which foods are high in fat and avoid them or eat them only occasionally.

FAT AND CALORIC CONTENT OF COOKED MEATS*

	Fat (grams)	Calories
Spareribs	35.0	396
Beef rib roast	21.0	285
Ground beef	17.1	263
Frankfurter (1)	15.7	176
T-bone steak	15.5	247
Lamb chop	11.9	223
Pork chop (loin cut)	11.3	250
Ham (rump cut)	10.8	205
Round steak	9.5	238
Veal cutlet	4.3	202
Ground beef, extra lean	3.9	163
Bacon (2 slices)	7.8	86

*3½ oz. cooked portion except where noted.

Nutrition Department; National Livestock and Meat Board — *The Nutritive Value of Meat* Chicago, 1976.

FAT AND CALORIC CONTENT OF DELI PRODUCTS

	Fat (grams)	Calories
Salami, 2 oz.	21.6	256
Bologna, 2 oz.	15.6	172
Liverwurst, 2 oz.	14.0	177
Summer sausage, 2 oz.	13.8	174
Broiled ham, 2 oz.	9.6	132
Turkey roll, 2 oz.	2.5	67

Try eating a leaner sandwich. Luncheon meats and hot dogs have more than 75 percent of their calories in the form of fat. Eat sliced breast of turkey or chicken, tuna, lean beef, or ham. Watch portion sizes. In contrast to bologna, turkey contains only 20 percent of its calories in the form of fat. By using plain yogurt or mustard instead of mayonnaise you can eliminate another 80 or more calories from fat. If you choose to eat high-fat luncheon meats, use one slice and some low-fat cheese instead of two or three slices of meat.

To further reduce fat in your diet, eat smaller meat portions. The following chart can help you estimate a 3-ounce cooked serving of meat, fish or poultry. Make it a goal to limit your total daily intake of meat, fish, poultry, eggs and cheese to 6 ounces or less.

PORTION SIZES OF FAT-CONTAINING FOODS
(Each equals 3 ounces)

1 piece **fish** (3×2½×½ inches)
1/2 medium breast of **chicken**
1 leg and 1 thigh of **chicken**
1/2 **Rock Cornish Hen**
One-quarter of one pound lean **ground beef** (one pound divided into 4 equal portions), each patty will be approximately 3 oz. when cooked.
1 slice lean **roast beef or ham** (3×3×3/4 inches)
1 medium **pork chop** (1/2 inch thick)
Approximately 10 medium **scallops** or **oysters**
12 medium **shrimp**
1 slice **pork** or calf **liver** (3×2¼×3/8 inches)
3/4 cup **chopped meat, fish** or **poultry**

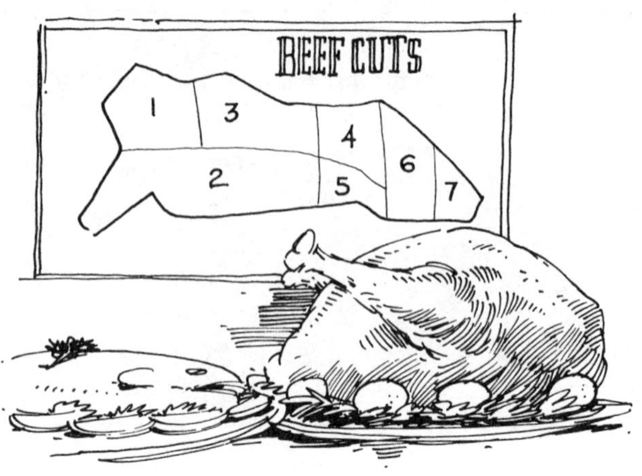

Meat Guide

Use Choices From this Group:

- *Beef*—choice or good grades, lean and well-trimmed chipped or dried, chuck, flank steak, lean ground beef, sirloin tip roast and steak, tenderloin, round, rump.
- *Veal*—all well-trimmed cuts (with the exception of the breast).
- *Pork*—leg (fresh ham), loin (rib or chopped), pork cubed steak, ribs, Canadian bacon,★ ham (center slices),★ ham (canned).★
- *Lamb*—leg, loin, shank, shoulder.
- *Luncheon meat*—commercially packaged thinly sliced lean beef, chicken, turkey or ham;★ turkey ham;★ turkey pastrami.★
- *Game*—pheasant, quail, rabbit, squirrel, venison.
- *Meat substitutes*—soybeans, dried beans, peas or lentils, soybean meat substitutes,★ tofu, peanut butter.

★High salt content

Decrease Choices From This Group:

- *Beef*—prime grade, brisket,★ corned beef,★ hamburger, pastrami,★ plate ribs, rib eye, heavily marbled meats.
- *Pork*—Boston, ground pork, loin back ribs, spareribs, bacon,★ salt pork,★ sausage,★ smoked pork shoulder, picnic★ or roll ham.
- *Lamb*—ground lamb, mutton.

- *Game*—duck, goose, venison sausage.
- ***Luncheon meat***—bologna,★ canned and packaged luncheon meats,★ frankfurters,★ head cheese, salami.★
- ***Miscellaneous***—commercially fried meat, fish, or poultry, meats canned or frozen in gravy or sauce.★

Shopping Tips

- Tenderness of meat is determined by: grade of meat; age of animal (younger animals are more tender); amount of fat or marbling (the more fat, the more tender); use of muscle (least used muscles are most tender). Leaner meats, which are not as tender, may require different cooking methods.
- Grading of meat is not based on food value, but on appearance. The amount of fat will be the major criterion in determining grade. Higher grade carcasses are more uniform in size, with a good intermingling of fat and a thick, firm fat covering; this meat will be juicier and more tender.

  Grades of Meats:
  USDA Prime
  USDA Choice
  USDA Good
  USDA Standard
  USDA Commercial

  Restaurants usually serve only prime grades of meat. Grocery stores generally carry choice grades as well as prime grades.
- Use the ***Meat Choice Continuum*** (page 59) to help identify low fat meats and lean cuts of meat.
- *Ground Beef:*
  When purchasing ground beef, select types as close to 10 percent fat as possible. Chopped sirloin or ground round makes the leanest ground beef, followed by very lean ground chuck.

  "Hamburger" or "chopped meat" has more than 25 percent fat. Regular hamburger may contain as much as 30 percent fat.

  Look for medium to deep color, which signifies a low fat content. (A light pink color is a warning that excess fat has been ground in with the meat.)

Regular ground beef costs less than lean and extra lean because it has more fat. You can remove a lot of fat from the regular ground beef by broiling or by breaking it up, cooking and draining it.

Lean and extra lean cost more but have less fat to begin with, so that after cooking you will end up with more cooked meat or a larger patty than with regular hamburger. After breaking up, cooking and draining, however, the fat content in regular, lean and extra lean is about the same.

- *Pork:*
  Many people erroneously believe that pork is high in fat. This is no longer true. Pork producers are now producing lean cuts of pork; lean pork chops and hams are examples.

  When choosing pork, look for lean cuts and those that are easy to trim. Sirloin roast, tenderloin and loin chops are good choices.

  Choose economical grades (choice and good) that are less marbled.

- *Frankfurters:*
  The term "all meat" may be misleading. According to USDA, such franks also contain ten percent water and five percent other ingredients (spices, flavorings, chemicals). Perhaps the label should say "all kinds of meat," for it includes muscle tissue from cattle, pigs and chickens with up to 30 percent of the natural fat. Thus, 45 percent of "all meat" frankfurters may be fat, water and additives.

  You'll also see the term "all beef." The difference is that the meat part will be derived from beef animals only. However, this does not translate as "all protein," since fat can also come from beef. The average frankfurter calorie sources are 80 percent fat and 12 percent protein.

  The simple frankfurter, which in addition to the meat products contains cereal, defatted wheat germ, and milk solids, is probably a better buy than the all meat or all beef franks. It contains only 2.5 percent less meat than all meat varieties and more nutrition in the long run. One pound of "all meat" frankfurters contains 1,343 calories and 59.4 grams of protein. One pound of frankfurters with cereal contains 1,124 calories and 65.3 grams of protein.

Cooking Tips

- Before cooking any type of meat, remove all visible fat. After cooking, remove any remaining fat.

- Baste meat with wine, tomato or lemon juice instead of drippings.
- Brown meats by broiling or cooking in non-stick pans with little or no oil. Instead of using butter or shortening to prevent sticking, use non-stick low-fat spray on frying and baking pans.
- Before making gravy or sauces, skim ice cubes through the drippings. Remove the congealed fat with a slotted spoon before mixing it with flour or cornstarch for gravies. Or use a gravy skimmer, or lay paper towels on the surface of the stock to absorb fat. For quick defatting, move pan off the heat. Fat will move toward the cooler area and can be skimmed off easily. Chill the stock overnight and lift off the hardened fat. This saves 100 calories per tablespoon of fat removed.
- To make gravies, use a cup or so of clear, defatted broth. In a jar, place 1 tablespoon of uncooked flour, or 1 to 2 tablespoons of browned flour for each 1/2 cup of liquid. Shake until smooth. Heat the remaining liquid in a saucepan, pour flour mixture into it and simmer, adding seasonings as desired. Flour can be browned to give the sauce a mahogany color if desired. This is done by placing flour in a shallow pan over low heat and stirring frequently, or by baking in an oven at 300 degrees for 15 minutes.
- Saute onions or other vegetables in water or broth instead of butter or oil, or cook for a few minutes in a microwave oven.
- Leaner (tougher) cuts of meat can be tenderized by three methods:

  1. Mechanical methods, such as cubing, grinding, pounding or thinly slicing across the grain.
  2. Acid methods, such as with marinade preparations. Marinades are composed of acids, oil, and herbs and spices. They need to contain an acid base which can be beer, wine, soy sauce, lemon juice, tomato juice, or vinegar.
  3. Slow cooking methods, such as by cooking slowly in liquids, stewing, pot roasting, and fricasseeing.

Meat Cooking Methods

- ***When roasting,*** use a rack so the meat will not soak in the fat that cooks out.
- ***When broiling,*** use a broiler pan so the fat drips away from the meat during cooking. (Covering the broiler pan with foil, however, will prevent fat from dripping into the bottom pan.) Placing water in the bottom of the broiler pan will prevent burned-on grease.

- *Charcoaling* refers to meat cooked on a rack over charcoal. This is another way to allow fat to drip away from meat while cooking.
- *Braising* refers to meat cooked in a covered pan on a rack. Cooking on a rack will also allow the fat to drip away.
- *When stewing and crock pot cooking,* skim fat off the broth.
- *Use frying minimally.* When frying, use oil for deep fat and pan frying. Oil used to fry vegetables may be reused. But oil used to fry beef, pork or chicken should be discarded, since the fat that cooks out of these meats is saturated and remains in the oil.
- *Batter frying* produces a very high fat product because batters absorb cooking fat. As an alternative, foods to be fried or deep fried may be dredged in flour or dipped in egg whites and then cracker meal. When cooked until done and not overdone, foods absorb only a minimal amount of oil. They will absorb excessive amounts only if immersed too long or if the oil is not hot enough. Corn oil is a good choice for deep fat frying because its smoking point is higher than other oils.

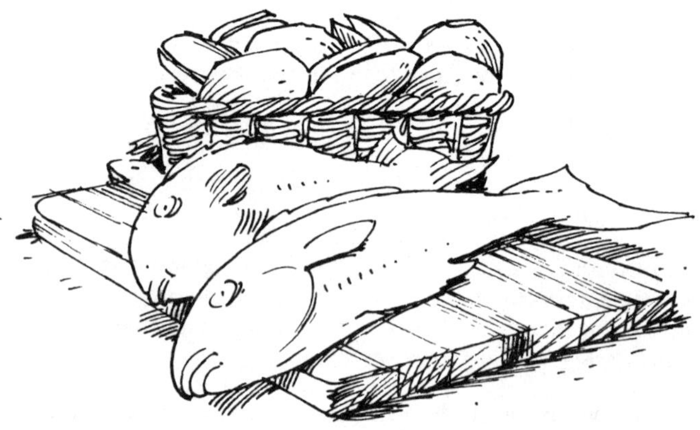

Fish

In 1980 Americans ate only one pound of fish and seafood for every ten pounds of beef and pork. Although consumption of beef and poultry has increased since the early 1900s, fish intake remains nearly the same. Poultry intake has increased the most dramatically—from 18 pounds per person per year in the early 1900s to 62 pounds per person per year in 1980—a 225 percent increase. Chicken alone accounted for approximately 80 percent of all poultry sales, which can probably be attributed to the popularity of chicken at fast-food restaurants.

This is surprising, for fish offers some real benefits: It is low in fat, high in nutrition and cooks quickly. In addition, there is a wide choice of taste and texture in fish and seafood. However, fish and seafood may be expensive, depending on the season and your location.

Fish contains a much greater percentage of polyunsaturated fat than do poultry and red meats, so it should be included in your menu frequently.

For years shellfish was regarded as being high in dietary cholesterol, but new analyses by the USDA indicate that older cholesterol tables were based on chemical analyses of foods that picked up non-cholesterol components along with cholesterol. As a result, many of the cholesterol values listed for shellfish were much too high. Shellfish are low in total fat and calories.

The newer analyses report that shellfish cholesterol values vary from 60 to 120 milligrams per 3 1/2 ounces. Even shrimp, the only shellfish thought to be higher in cholesterol, may have as low as 90 milligrams of cholesterol for a 3 1/2-ounce cooked portion. Older values were over 150 milligrams.

Not only does eating more of most kinds of fish offer a way to cut back on cholesterol, fat and calories, but fish rich in certain oils may also help to prevent heart attacks. These special polyunsaturated oils, which are different from those of vegetable origin, are called omega-3 fatty acids—technically named eicosapentaenoic acid (EPA) and docosahexaenoic acid (DHA). All fish and shellfish contain them, but oilier, fattier fish are the richest sources of omega-3 fatty acids. Fish with the highest concentration of EPA come from cold, deepwater habitats. The EPA acts as an antifreeze in the cold water, enabling a fish's cells to remain flexible. EPA's ability to keep a fish's fat from hardening is important to fish swimming in cold water. Medium to high fat fish have the highest concentration of EPA. This includes salmon, albacore, bluefish tuna, mackerel, sablefish, herring, rainbow trout and whitefish. Many specialists recommend eating at least two fish meals a week to benefit from the effects of EPA in the diet.

A number of studies have shown that eating large amounts of omega-3 fatty acids can decrease the tendency of blood platelet cells, involved with clotting, to stick or clump together. This decreases the likelihood of forming clots that can block blood flow to the heart and result in a heart attack. Omega-3 fatty acids have also been shown to lower blood triglyceride and cholesterol levels, and reduce blood pressure.

The omega-3 fatty acid research began more than ten years ago when it was discovered that Greenland Eskimos and Japanese fishermen who eat large amounts of fish have a surprisingly low incidence of heart attacks. This area of research is continuing but there is not yet enough evidence to know how to apply this information. The best bet is to increase your intake of omega-3 fatty acids by eating reasonable portions of all types of fish several times a week. Long-term effects of eating large quantities of fish oil are not known, so fish oil supplements should be avoided. You should be particularly careful of cod liver oil, which can be toxic in high doses.

Fish can be divided into lean and fat fish. However, even high fat fish are lower in total fat and cholesterol than most cuts of meat as well as containing polyunsaturated fat along with omega-3 fatty acids.

- ***Lean Fish:*** Bluefish, cod (torsk), carp, crappie, flounder, grouper, haddock, lake herring, hake, halibut, ocean perch, pollock, walleyed pike, yellow perch, red snapper, sea bass, sole, swordfish, whiting, striped bass (rockfish).
- ***Fat Fish:*** Butterfish, mackerel, pompano, porgie, salmon, herring, striped bass, tuna, lake trout, whitefish, rainbow trout, eel, catfish, mullet, sablefish, anchovies, canned sardines, smelt.

The following are examples of the fat and calories per serving of different types of fish:

FAT AND CALORIC CONTENT OF 3½ OUNCES COOKED FISH

	Fat (grams)	Calories
Shrimp	1.1	116
Walleyed Pike	1.2	93
Lobster	1.9	91
Crabmeat	2.1	86
Cod (Torsk)	5.3	168
Salmon steak	7.4	182
Trout, Brook	11.2	196
Herring, smoked	12.4	196
Tuna, water-packed	0.8	126
Tuna, oil-packed	20.3	285

Fish and Shellfish Guide

Increase Choices From This Group:

- All freshwater and saltwater fish, clams, crab, scallops, lobster, oyster, salmon and tuna (drain the oil). Water-packed tuna contains one percent fat in comparison to the 21 percent fat in oil-packed tuna.

Decrease Choices From This Group:

- Caviar, eel, frozen breaded fish.

Shopping Tips

The following are signs of fresh fish:

Eyes are bright and bulging.
No fishy smell; smells fresh.
Shiny, resilient skin that springs back when pressed with a finger.
Gills are bright.
Skin is free of slime; flesh is firm and moist.
Filets are held together tightly and are not dry or curled at the edges.

Newly-purchased fish should be washed, patted dry and covered with an air-tight wrapper. Fish can be stored in a refrigerator for up to two days or in a freezer for up to three months.

Cooking Tips

Lean fish tastes great poached, steamed or in chowders. But no matter which method you choose, remember: ***DON'T OVERCOOK.*** Overcooked fish is dry and tough. Fish should be cooked only enough to coagulate (set) the protein; then it will be moist and tender. Looking at the fish will help you determine when it is ready. As soon as it loses its translucence and becomes opaque, the protein is set. The best way to judge is by fork-testing. Remove it from the heat as soon as it flakes easily when poked with a fork.

- ***Low temperatures*** are best for most fish cookery, with the exception of frying. The important point is to adjust the time according to the temperature. Cooking fish requires close attention, but only for 10 to 15 minutes. Cook fish 10 minutes for each one-inch thickness at the thickest part. Double time for frozen fish. Exceptions are deep frying and microwaving. Microwave fish fillets 3 minutes per pound.

- ***Oven cooking*** requires the least attention, is simple to do and easy to clean up. To bake, preheat your oven to 350. Season fish lightly and place in a greased baking dish. Brush with a little oil. Add a little lemon juice and grated onion for flavor. Bake in a moderate oven (350) about 20 to 25 minutes. Give it the fork test for doneness. If a sauce is desired, vegetable broth, tomato sauce or skim milk can be added to just cover the fish before baking.

- ***Broiling*** is the quickest, simplest method of cooking fish. Season fish as desired. Grease the broiler pan. Place the fish directly on the broiler pan and brush with oil or French dressing. Insert the pan so the top of the fish is two or three inches from the heat and broil 10 to 15 minutes. Thinner pieces may be done quickly and need not be turned. Thick pieces cook more evenly and will be delicately browned if turned halfway through cooking.

- ***When poaching,*** wrap the fish in a piece of cheesecloth. This will make it easier to lift from the pot when it's done and will minimize breaking. Heat your chosen poaching liquid in a deep skillet, using enough liquid to just cover the fish. Skim milk, vegetable bouillon, tomato juice or lightly salted water all work well. Place whole fish fillets in the liquid and adjust heat so the liquid is barely simmering. Cover the skillet and cook until fish flakes easily with a fork, about 5 to 10 minutes.

- ***Steaming*** fish results in a smaller amount of nutrient loss than submerging it in a liquid (poaching or simmering). When steaming fish, place it on an ovenproof plate or rack above simmering or boiling water; never submerge it. Cover. The steam circulates around the fish, thus cooking it gently. Fish steamers are expensive, but can be improvised. Use a wok with an ovenproof plate or a roasting pan with a rack. Cover it with a lid. To prevent fish from falling apart, wrap it in cheesecloth and handle it very gently while cooking.

- ***Frying*** is the least preferred method of preparing fish, since it adds unnecessary fats. Those who long for the crisp crust and browned flavor will find that **oven frying** is the answer—it requires much less fat. Dip the pieces of fish into seasoned skim milk and roll in fine dry bread crumbs. To heighten color, add a teaspoon of paprika to each cup of bread crumbs. Arrange the coated pieces side by side in a well-greased baking dish. Drizzle a small amount of oil over the fish—about 2 tablespoons per pound. Place in a very hot oven (500) for 10 to 15 minutes.

- ***Flavor*** fish with lemon juice, dill weed, parsley, oregano, basil, thyme, marjoram, bay leaf, onion and garlic powder, tarragon, or paprika. Use 1/4 teaspoon of one or two herbs or spices per pound of seafood. To substitute dry herbs for fresh herbs, use 1/3 teaspoon powdered or 1/2 teaspoon crushed dry herbs for every tablespoon of fresh chopped herbs.

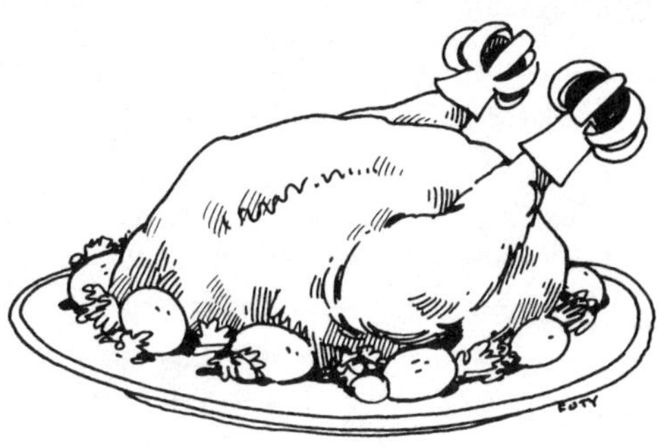

Poultry

The advantages of poultry are many. Besides being a good source of nutrients, poultry is lower in fats and calories than most meats. Its flavors blend well with many foods and seasonings. It can be served at different temperatures and in many forms (soups, salads, entrees). In addition, it is economical.

Chicken and turkey contain less saturated fat than beef, pork and lamb. Most of the fat in poultry is concentrated just beneath the skin, so it should be removed before eating. For example, a chicken breast roasted without the skin has 4 grams of fat per 4 ounce serving with 19 percent of the calories from fat; roasted with the skin it has 9 grams of fat per 4 ounce serving with 36 percent of the calories from fat.

Chicken thighs roasted without the skin have 12 grams of fat per 4 ounce serving with 47 percent of the total calories from fat; roasted with the skin they have 18 grams of fat per 4 ounce serving with 57 percent of the total calories from fat. Extra crispy, Kentucky Fried Chicken with skin will have 24 to 25 grams of fat per 4 ounce serving with 56 to 61 percent of the total calories from fat.

Poultry Guide

Increase Choices From This Group:

Chicken, rock cornish game hens, turkey, quail, wild duck, pheasant.

Decrease Choices From This Group:

Poultry skin, domestic duck, goose, capon, turkey and chicken franks.

Shopping Tips

- When choosing whole turkeys, avoid self-basters. These are usually injected with saturated fats.
- Duck and goose are usually high in fat. One pound of domestic duck has 1,215 calories and 109 grams of fat, while a pound of chicken has 385 calories and 15 grams of fat! However, wild duck is lower in calories and fat than domestic duck.
- Signs of quality in poultry are: full body (especially around the breast), meaty legs, no odor and moderate amounts of fat.
- To store raw poultry, wash and wrap it in a clean, airtight package and place it in the coldest part of the refrigerator. Use within two days. Defrost poultry in the refrigerator rather than at room temperature.

Cooking Tips

- Use seasonings such as lemon juice, tomatoes, herbs or wines rather than high fat and calorie extras such as butter or sour cream.
- For a quick "Shake and Bake," moisten chicken with skim milk or water and then dip it into cracker crumbs in a paper bag. Bake as usual in a greased shallow pan in a 350-degree oven for 45-60 minutes.
- Chicken can be cooked with the skin on or off. The important thing is to remove the skin before eating. If broiling chicken with the skin off, first sprinkle a few ice chips over the chicken. This will broil the chicken more rapidly and help keep it moist.

MEAT CHOICE CONTINUUM*

- Leanest cuts, trimmed
- Broiled, unless otherwise specified
- No butter or other fat added in cooking

Contains the least amount of saturated fat and cholesterol ⟵⟶ **Contains the greatest amount of saturated fat and cholesterol**

clams plain **scallops** plain **oysters** plain	**fish** white	**fish** pink	**shrimp** plain	**chicken** light w/o skin **turkey** light w/o skin **lobster** w/o butter **scallops** fried **oysters** fried **fish** fried fillets	**chicken** dark w/o skin	**venison**	**turkey** dark w/o skin	**veal** loin **beef** round steak **beef** flank steak **beef** sirloin tip **beef** cube steak **beef** arm pot roast **pork** center ham slice	**beef** sirloin **beef** t-bone **beef** porterhouse **beef** rump roast **beef** lean stew meat **beef** loin	**hamburger** lean	**beef** prime rib	**hamburger** regular	**liver** beef or calf **luncheon meats** bologna frank- furters salami

*Adapted from MRFITT Minneapolis
Clinical Center Nutrition Education Material.

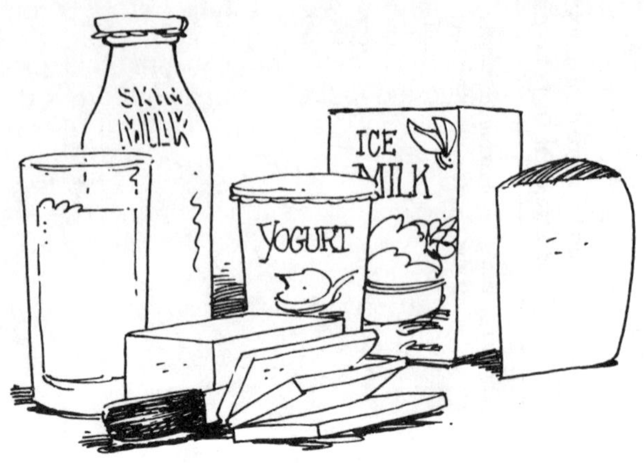

Dairy Products

Milk is an excellent source of protein, calcium, B vitamins and fat soluble vitamins A and D. (A fat-soluble vitamin is one that is carried by fat in food and stored with fat in the body.) Skim milk and nonfat dry milk lose fat-soluble vitamins as fat is removed in processing, but vitamin A and D enriched products are readily available and make nonfat milk every bit as nutritionally complete as whole milk. Other minerals plentiful in milk include phosphorus, potassium and sodium.

Cow's milk contains nearly all the nutrients needed to maintain life and support growth. In addition, milk protein complements grain and vegetable proteins. Thus, milk in your cereal bowl improves the protein value of your cereal.

Though it is easy to digest compared with other animal fats, milk fat is 65 percent saturated fatty acids and only 4 percent polyunsaturated fatty acids. Low fat products offer reduced levels of fat and cholesterol, as well as fewer calories.

Lactose, also known as milk sugar, is what gives cow's milk its sweet taste. Lactose is the main carbohydrate in milk, providing 30 to 50 percent of its calories. However, lactose must be chemically converted in the body so it can be digested. An enzyme called lactase does the converting. Most people have enough lactase in their digestive system to complete the task.

Some people have trouble digesting lactose and are considered lactose intolerant. Lactose-reduced milk products are available in some areas, and lactase, the enzyme for converting lactose, can be purchased at some pharmacies. True lactase enzyme is usually sold in a bottle. Four or five drops of the enzyme are added to a quart of milk. The milk is stirred or shaken and left in a refrigerator for 24 hours, and approximately 70 percent of the lactose is converted.

When people with a lactase deficiency consume milk products, the lactose remains undigested in the intestine and causes diarrhea, gas, bloating, abdominal pain and/or cramps. This is a fairly common problem, particularly in non-Caucasians.

Some individuals can tolerate aged cheese and cottage cheese better than non-fermented dairy products. Even though yogurt has a fairly high lactose content, studies have shown that the bacteria used to make yogurt produce the enzyme lactase, which breaks down about 25 percent of the lactose.

By the time the yogurt gets to the grocery store, it has become quite acidic and is chilled, which causes the bacteria to stop breaking down the lactose. When the yogurt is eaten, the warmth of the body and the low acid conditions of the small intestine allow the bacteria to again produce lactase.

All things considered, low-fat milk products are a triple bonus: 1)fewer calories, 2) less saturated fat, and 3) less cholesterol—all without losing the other valuable nutrients found in whole milk. (Children below the age of 2 should be kept on whole milk to make sure they get enough fat to provide essential fatty acids.)

COMPARE:

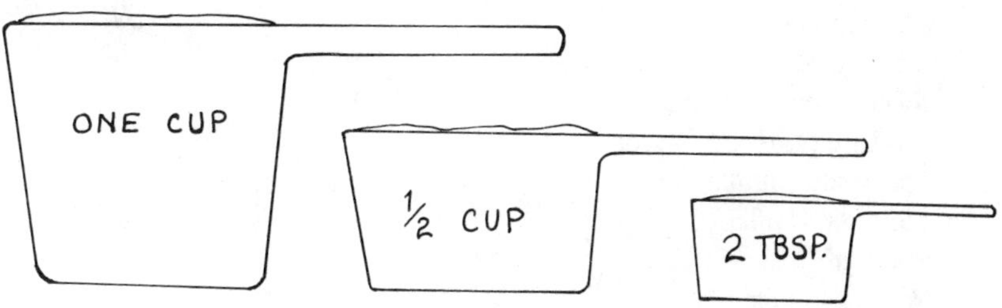

1 cup low-fat yogurt = 1/2 cup sour cream = 2 Tbsp. mayonnaise
Each of the above amounts contains 100 calories.

The following table lists the grams of fat and calories found in dairy products:

FAT AND CALORIC CONTENT OF DAIRY PRODUCTS

	Fat (grams)	Calories
Milk (8 oz. serving):		
Skim milk	0.5	90
Buttermilk	2.2	100
1% milk	2.0	100
2% milk	4.6	120
Whole milk	8.1	150
Chocolate milk*	8.5	210
Yogurt (8 oz. serving):		
Low-fat plain	3.4	130
Low-fat with fruit*	3.0	260
Whole milk yogurt	7.0	150
Cream (1 Tbsp.)		
Half and half	1.7	20
Sour cream	2.5	25
Whipping cream	4.6	45
Nondairy creamer	3.0	33
Cottage Cheese (½ cup):		
2% creamed	2.0	100
4% creamed	5.1	120
Ricotta cheese (1 oz.)	3.0	45
Frozen dairy products (½ cup):		
Ice cream, vanilla	7.2	140
Ice milk, vanilla	2.8	90
Sherbet**	1.7	130
Yogurt, vanilla	1.0	70
Yogurt, fruit flavor**	1.0	108

*High sugar content.

**The calories from fat are relatively low in these desserts, but their sugar content raises the total number of calories.

Shopping Tips

- To achieve positive changes in your eating habits, consider substituting low fat products for the following dairy items:
  Whole milk
  Half and half
  Chocolate milk
  Nondairy coffee creamers
  Cheese made from whole milk or cream
  Butter
  Ice cream
  Cream cheese
  Whipped toppings
  Condensed milk
  Sour cream
  Whipped cream

  Purchase and use dairy products that are lower in fat:

  Skim or nonfat milk
  Low-fat milk
  Nonfat dried milk
  Low-fat yogurt
  Buttermilk (made from skim milk)
  Cottage cheese
  Low-fat or skim milk cheese (without added cream)
  Evaporated skim milk

- If you presently drink whole milk, make changes gradually. Try using 2% milk for a few weeks, then 1% milk and eventually skim milk.

- Check to be sure that the skim milk and nonfat dry milk you purchase are vitamin A and D enriched.

- Imitation creams, such as coffee whiteners, are nondairy products—but nondairy does not mean nonfat. They are usually made from coconut and palm oil, which are highly saturated fats. And they contain corn syrup, emulsifiers (fats added to make the liquid creamy), and artificial flavoring. If you are going to use a creamer, you might as well buy the real thing! Try using instant nonfat dry milk powder or skim milk in your coffee as a healthful alternative.

- Avoid filled milk or imitation milk that uses vegetable fat to replace the butterfat. Coconut oil is the typical fat in these products.

- Fruit flavored brands of yogurt rely on imitation flavoring and coloring. All contain refined sugar. Fruit flavored yogurt is not a good low-calorie lunch: 1 cup frequently has between 250 and 280 calories, of which only 100 to 125 calories come from the yogurt. The other calories come from added sugar (six teaspoons) or fruit syrups. As an alternative, buy some fruit to enhance plain yogurt, and then sit down to a low-fat, low-calorie lunch.

- Ice milks and frozen yogurt are low-calorie desserts. The better choices will have less than 2 percent fat and a caloric content under 100 per half-cup serving.

Cooking Tips

- Substituting skim milk, buttermilk, yogurt or real fruit juices for whole milk or cream is a positive step toward making your favorite dairy product lower in fat, cholesterol and calories without sacrificing quality.

- Plain, unflavored yogurt can be the most versatile food in your kitchen. Like sweet and sour cream, it adds lightness to baked goods, but not excess fat and calories. Whenever a recipe calls for cream—sweet or sour—substitute an equal amount of yogurt. Yogurt can even replace cream and milk in quiches, stews, salad dressings, sauces, custard, etc. Two tablespoons of yogurt contain only 16 calories, compared with 50 calories in 2 tablespoons of sour cream and 200 calories in 2 tablespoons of mayonnaise! If yogurt is watery, drain it in a strainer lined with cheesecloth before using.

- To prevent yogurt from separating during cooking, mix 1 tablespoon of cornstarch with a tablespoon of yogurt and stir this into 1 cup of yogurt. Continue stirring over medium heat until thickened, or whenever possible, add yogurt to cooked foods after removing from the heat source.

- Need a good dip for a party? Try adding onion and garlic powder or a salad dressing mix to plain yogurt. Yogurt can also replace sour cream or a large portion of the mayonnaise in your favorite dip recipes. Choose a firm yogurt for the best consistency.

- To make a sour cream substitute, blend a cup of 1% milkfat cottage cheese with a tablespoon of skim milk. Add lemon juice to taste.

- When you substitute skim or nonfat dry milk in cooking, add a drop of vanilla extract per cup to make the cream soup or custard taste richer still.

- Nonfat dry milk powder can become rancid if allowed to stand in your cupboard for too long. During warm weather, keep opened boxes in your refrigerator.
- Evaporated skim milk can be used in recipes that call for evaporated milk. It can also be whipped when partially frozen.
- To make a low-fat, low-calorie whipped topping, try one of the following:
  1. Whip together 2 egg whites and 1/2 teaspoon cream of tartar. Whip in 2 to 3 tablespoons sugar with 1/2 cup part-skim ricotta cheese. Fold in the egg whites and refrigerate until served. Yield: one cup (10 servings). One serving has 34 calories and 1 gram fat (and is a 1/3 skim milk exchange if you are on an exchange meal plan).
  2. Combine 1/2 cup of nonfat dry milk powder and 1/2 cup of water in a chilled bowl. Beat with an electric or rotary beater until soft peaks form (approximately 5 minutes). Add 2 tablespoons of orange juice and 2 tablespoons of honey, maple syrup or sugar and continue beating until fluffy (about five minutes). Keep refrigerated until needed and use within two hours.
- To make low-fat white sauce, follow the instructions below. The thickness of the sauce depends upon the amount of flour per cup of liquid and not the liquid that is used. You will want a different degree of thickness depending on how the sauce is to be used.

WHITE SAUCES OF VARYING THICKNESSES

Desired Thickness	Amount of Liquid (Skim Milk)	Amount of Flour	Amount of Margarine
Thin sauce (use over vegetables)	1 cup	1 Tbsp.	1 Tbsp.
Medium sauce (use with pasta, potato dishes, etc.)	1 cup	2 Tbsp.	2 Tbsp.
Thick sauce (use in souffles, in place of cream soup)	1 cup	3 Tbsp.	3 Tbsp.

Melt the margarine. It is important to fully cook the flour for at least two minutes to eliminate any raw, starchy taste. Stir it constantly over medium heat to prevent sticking or browning, which gives the sauce a grayish appearance. The sauce should remain white. Using cornstarch in place of flour will give the sauce a different taste, appearance and viscosity. Be sure to use skim milk.

Some recipes do not require making a sauce or paste of fat and flour or cornstarch. The main thing is to separate the starch granules from each other so they don't form lumps. This can be accomplished by adding cold milk directly to the flour or cornstarch and not using any fat. Once smoothly blended, stir the starch-liquid mixture constantly over medium heat until it boils.

Cheese

Cheese generally provides more fat than does an equal portion of cooked meat, and the fat is mostly saturated. Cholesterol is also found in cheese. The one exception is cottage cheese, which is also lower in fat. People on vegetarian diets should be cautious of using cheese extensively as a protein source, because it has a high content of fat and cholesterol. A few ounces of cheese a day should be your upper limit.

We recommend that everyone limit intake of hard and processed cheeses. When using cheese, substitute 1 ounce of cheese for 1 ounce of red meat in your diet.

FAT, SATURATED FAT, CALORIC, AND SODIUM CONTENT OF VARIOUS CHEESES

	Total Fat (grams)	Saturated Fat (grams)	Calories	Sodium (milligrams)
Mozzarella, part skim, 1 oz.	4.8	3.1	80	150
Cheese food, 1 oz.	7.0	4.3	90	320
Swiss, 1 oz.	7.8	5.0	110	75
Parmesan, grated, 1 oz.	8.5	5.4	130	530
Monterey Jack, 1 oz.	8.6	5.3	110	150
American, processed, 1 oz.	8.9	5.6	110	405
Cheddar, 1 oz.	9.4	6.0	110	175
Cream cheese, 1 oz.	9.9	6.2	100	85

Cheese Guide

Fat content of cheese is specified in two ways: grams of fat per ounce of cheese, or percent of fat (grams of fat per 100 grams, or approximately 3 1/2 ounces of cheese). The following categories should help you make selections.

- Cheeses with 1 to 2 grams of fat per ounce come primarily from skim milk.

  Examples:
  - Low-fat cottage cheese (2%)
  - Regular cottage cheese (4%)
  - Chef's Delight★
  - Diet cheeses:
    - Calorie Wise (Kraft) cheese spread★
    - Countdown (Fisher)★
    - Light 'n Lively American pasteurized process cheese (Kraft)★
    - Lite-Line (Borden)★
    - Weight Watchers low-fat cheese slices★
  - Farmer's
  - Gammelost (Norwegian strong)
  - Hoop cheese
  - Laughing Cow skim milk cheese wedges (3/4 oz.)
  - May Bud skim milk (Purity)
  - Pot cheese
  - Ricotta, made with part skim milk
  - Sap Sago
  - St. Otho
  - Wisconsin Skim Milk Cheese (Purity)

  ★High Sodium Content.

- Cheeses with 3 to 5 grams of fat per ounce should be used in place of meat, not in addition to it. The saturated fat and cholesterol content of those cheeses are similar to 1 ounce of lean meat.

  Examples:
  - Cheez Whiz cheese spread
  - Cheriss (similar to Baby Swiss)
  - Feta
  - Green River skim milk cheese (Lucerne)
  - Mozzarella, part skim
  - Mozzarella, pizza (Kraft)
  - Neufchatel
  - Olympia diet cheese
  - Parmesan cheese used in small amounts
  - Philadelphia Light (Kraft) cream cheese
  - Ricotta, whole milk
  - Skim American (Borden)

Slimline (Borden)
Slimost Lowfat Colby
Tivoli Danalette (a low-fat Danbo cheese)
Weight Watchers natural part skim milk cheese

- Cheeses with 6 to 8 grams of low cholesterol fat per pound (filled skim milk cheese) are similar in total fat to regular cheese but low in cholesterol and saturated fat. Select filled cheese made with corn, cottonseed, safflower or sunflower seed oils.

  Examples:
  Cheezola (Fisher), corn oil, cholesterol free★
  Dorman's Low-chol or Tilsiter cheese
  Hickory Farms, Longhorn Lyte
  Hickory Farms, Smokey Lyte★
  Lorraine Swiss
  Merrywood Farm's Nu Trend cheeses:
  Caraway Snack
  Onion Snack
  Hot 'N Spicy
  Mild 'N Mellow
  Hickory Smoked
  Mini-Cholesterol
  Scandic Cholesterol Free Cheese
  ★High Sodium Content.

- Cheeses with 6 to 8 grams of fat per ounce are made from whole milk. They contain a large amount of saturated fat and cholesterol.

  Examples:
  Brick
  Cheddar
  Colby
  Monterey Jack
  Swiss

- Cheeses with 9 to 11 grams of fat per ounce are made from whole milk with added butterfat (milk fat). They are high fat cheeses that contain up to a tablespoon of fat per ounce.

  Examples:
  Cream cheese
  Brie

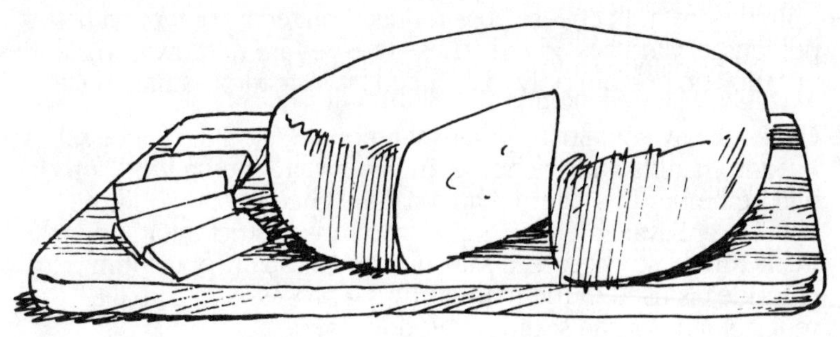

Shopping Tips

- Check the labels on cheese. If the fat content is listed, it should be indicated in grams of fat per ounce or in percent of fat [grams of fat per 100 grams (3 1/2 oz.) of cheese].
- Avoid purchasing natural cheeses containing more than 9 percent butterfat or 6 or more grams of fat per ounce. Cheeses that contain more than 20 percent fat are the highest in butterfat.

  Examples of varieties to avoid are:
  - Natural cheeses, such as cheddar, brick, colby, Swiss
  - Processed cheeses
  - Cream cheese
- Processed cheeses, cheese foods, and cheese spreads are high in sodium. If you must choose a processed form, look for a product labeled "low sodium."
- Hard cheeses are often sold unlabeled. Or they may be labeled "made from partially skimmed milk" with no further information about fat or caloric content. Many of these cheeses offer no significant reduction in fat or calories. Many hard cheeses made from partially skimmed milk have additional butterfat added.
- Soft, part skim milk cheeses, such as mozzarella and ricotta, are lower in fat and calories than hard cheese. Feta cheese and Neufchatel cheese are also somewhat lower in fat and caloric content.
- Cheese must be labeled "imitation cheese" if it contains less butterfat than required by the official standards for cheese. As an example, a cheddar that is identical to other cheddars except that it contains less fat must be labeled "imitation," even though it may have more protein than the so-called real cheddar.

- "Filled skim milk cheese" has reduced butterfat content with polyunsaturated fats added. These cheeses are not lower in calories but they do contain polyunsaturated fat instead of saturated fats.

- Cheeses may contain a significant amount of sodium, since salt is used in manufacturing cheese. In general, a "cheese food" product will be higher in sodium than a natural cheese. Low-sodium cheeses are available for people who must restrict their sodium intake. In these cheeses, a salt substitute (usually potassium chloride) is used in the manufacturing process as a partial replacement for the sodium chloride.

Cooking Tips

Perhaps you don't consider low-fat cheeses to be good "eating" cheeses. Chances are you probably won't be able to tell the difference when using them in the preparation of cheese sauces, grated cheese toppings or in casseroles.

- Using a mixture of low-fat cheese with mozzarrela on a pizza makes a cheese that has 2 grams of fat per ounce rather than the usual 4 grams.

- Use small amounts of freshly grated Parmesan for a cheese flavor topping. One tablespoon is very light and contains only 1.5 grams of fat and 23 calories.

Fats, Oils, Nuts and Seeds

There are other sources of fat in the diet in addition to meats, fish, poultry and dairy products. Some examples are oils, margarines, baked goods, coconut, avocado, milk chocolate and cream soups. The table on page 72 gives you information about the type of fat and number of calories in various fats and oils.

Safflower oil is the vegetable oil that is the highest in polyunsaturated fatty acids (74 percent) and lowest in saturated fatty acids (9 percent). By comparison, corn oil has 58 percent polyunsaturated and 13 percent saturated fatty acids.

Ever wondered where safflower oil comes from? Safflower is a thistle-like plant that originated in ancient India. Virtually all safflower oil prepared in the United States comes from fields in California or Montana. Safflower is very hardy and drought-resistant and grows best in drier climates.

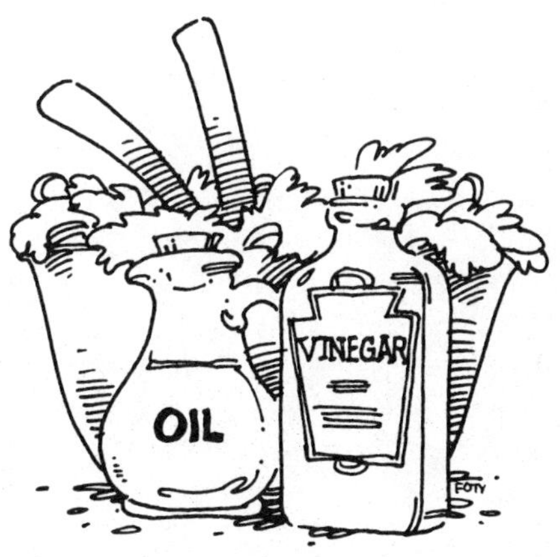

Nuts and seeds can also contribute significant amounts of protein, vegetable fats and therefore calories to the diet. Consequently, you should not eat many nuts if on a low-calorie diet. Nuts (54 percent fat by weight) have a lot of energy—170 to 190 calories per ounce. However, the type of fat found in nuts and seeds is unsaturated or monounsaturated. Eating dry roasted nuts lowers the fat content only a little. The majority of the fat calories are contained within the nut, not added in the roasting process.

Protein from plant sources is desirable because it is accompanied by little saturated fat and no cholesterol. One ounce of nuts supplies about 10 percent of the RDA for protein. However, this is not a complete protein and must be combined with either grains, legumes or milk products to equal the protein quality of meat. In comparison,

TYPE OF FAT AND NUMBER OF CALORIES IN FATS AND OILS

	Percent Poly-Unsaturated Fat	Percent Saturated Fat	Percent Mono-Unsaturated Fat	Calories Per Tbsp.
FATS AND OILS				
Safflower oil	75%	11%	14%	125
Sunflower oil	61%	11%	28%	125
Soybean oil	61%	14%	25%	125
Corn oil	57%	14%	29%	125
Cottonseed oil	46%	29%	25%	125
Olive oil	28%	21%	51%	125
Peanut oil	14%	14%	72%	125
Palm oil	2%	81%	17%	125
Coconut oil	2%	86%	12%	125
TUB MARGARINES				
Liquid safflower oil	63%	14%	23%	100
Liquid corn oil	49%	18%	33%	100
STICK MARGARINES				
Liquid corn oil	38%	19%	43%	100
Partially hydrogenated	19%	23%	58%	100
Imitation (diet) margarine	50%	20%	30%	50
MAYONNAISE	60%	20%	20%	100
SHORTENING	25%	25%	50%	100
LARD	8%	42%	50%	115
CHICKEN FAT	26%	29%	45%	125
BEEF FAT	4%	48%	48%	125
BUTTER	trace	60%	40%	100

a 1 ounce serving of meat supplies about 13 percent of the RDA for protein.

Most nuts will keep for up to 12 months under proper storage conditions. You must prevent them from picking up moisture. Do not store nuts with any item that has a strong odor, such as fresh fruits, onions, potatoes or meat. Packaged nuts will hold up well in room temperatures and should be stored in cool, dry places if they are to be held for any length of time.

FAT AND CALORIC CONTENT OF NUTS AND SEEDS

	Fat (grams)	Calories
Almonds, ¼ cup, 1 oz.	16.2	176
Cashews, ¼ cup, 1 oz.	13.8	168
Peanuts, ¼ cup, 1 oz.	14.0	162
Peanut butter, 2 Tbsp.	16.1	90
Pumpkin seeds, ¼ cup, 1 oz.	13.3	158
Sunflower seeds, kernels, ¼ cup, 1 oz.	13.5	160
Walnuts, ¼ cup, 1 oz.	19.4	196

Fats and Oils Guide

Use Choices From This Group:

Margarines (liquid vegetable oil should be the first ingredient, but some hardening oil or hydrogenation is necessary in margarines, otherwise they would be too soft). Tub or soft margarines (liquid oil should be the first ingredient).
Liquid vegetable oils—corn, cottonseed, sesame, soybean, sunflower, safflower.
Salad dressings and mayonnaise made from polyunsaturated oils.

Decrease Choices From This Group:

Butter
Coconut oil
Lard
Palm kernel oil
Salt pork
Completely hydrogenated margarines and shortenings
Sour Cream
Peanut oil and olive oil—use only occasionally for flavor

Shopping Tips

- *Read labels:* If the only fat listed on the label is "hydrogenated" or "hardened" oil, then the oil has been completely saturated.

  If the label states "liquid vegetable oil, partially hydrogenated," then there are more unsaturated than saturated fats present.

  If the order is reversed and the partially hydrogenated oil appears before the liquid, then there are more saturated fats.

- ***The American Heart Association*** has three categories for classifying both margarines and oils: preferred, acceptable, and not recommended.

  1. Preferred choices are products containing 100 percent safflower, corn, soy, cottonseed, or a mixture of these oils. Sesame seed oil and sunflower seed oil are also preferred. However, these oils are not usually available and are expensive.

  2. An acceptable choice is soybean oil that has been "specially processed," which means it has been partially hydrogenated.

  3. Not recommended for general use are peanut and olive oils, since they are monounsaturated fats. Small amount may be used for flavor. Food products containing "vegetable oil" or "vegetable fat" usually are made from coconut, palm kernel or other plant oils. They do not contain polyunsaturated fat and should be avoided.

- The phrases "nondairy," "contains no animal fat," or "vegetable fat" do not necessarily imply that a product is low in total fat or in saturated fat. It may be quite high in fat or contain coconut oil or palm oil, both of which are saturated fats.

- ***Tub margarine*** made from liquid unsaturated oil is 50 to 60 percent polyunsaturated, while stick margarines made from liquid unsaturated oils are only about 40 percent polyunsaturated.

- ***Diet margarine*** contains half the calories of regular margarine and butter, because half of the fat content has been replaced with water. Still, it has 50 calories per tablespoon.

- ***Choose a low-calorie or a low-fat salad dressing*** that has less than 16 calories per tablespoon. Or, when using regular salad dressing, use it sparingly. Instead of pouring it on, place a small amount in a separate dish and just wet your fork with it before you insert it in each bite of salad.

- ***Low-fat hot cocoa or milkshake mixes*** should be made with nonfat milk powder.

Cooking Tips

- ***Use liquid vegetable oils whenever possible.*** Use polyunsaturated oils for salad dressings, marinating meats, basting, browning, sauteeing, deep fat frying, pan frying, and in recipes calling for shortening. If a recipe calls for 1 cup of hardened shortening, use 3/4 cup of liquid vegetable oil; for 1/2 cup of shortening, use 1/3 cup of vegetable oil.
- If you leave out the nuts when making your favorite quick bread or cookies, you will save 50 calories or more in fat per serving. Or try finely chopping a few nuts and sprinkling them on top.
- Commercial mayonnaise and salad dressings are almost all pure fat—from 85 to 98 percent of total calories are fat. Low-calorie dressings sold in stores do help cut about 50 fat calories per serving. But a homemade, low-fat dressing such as yogurt and dill, or lemon and tomato juice with herbs, can have less than 20 calories per serving.
- ***Here's a trick to try with your favorite mayonnaise dressing or with sour cream recipes:*** Replace half to three fourths of the mayonnaise (100 calories per tablespoon) or sour cream (25 calories per tablespoon) with plain yogurt (8 calories per tablespoon).
- ***When a recipe calls for butter or solid shortening,*** use a stick margarine.
- ***For 1 square (1 ounce) of chocolate,*** use 2 to 3 Tbsp. cocoa plus 1 Tbsp. margarine or oil.
- ***Keep seeds such as sesame and sunflower on hand;*** you will find endless uses for them. Use raw nuts and seeds when cooking, but for other purposes, enhance the flavor by light toasting. Toast seeds and nuts at 300 degrees and stir them often.
- ***You can make nut and seed butters.*** Put nuts or seeds in a dry blender jar, just 1/4 cup at a time, and blend at high speed for a few seconds. Turn off the blender and stir the mixture. Repeat until the meal is uniformly ground. To make nut butter, mix a small amount of oil into the meal. Start with 1 tablespoon per cup of meal and gradually add more until it reaches the desired consistency.

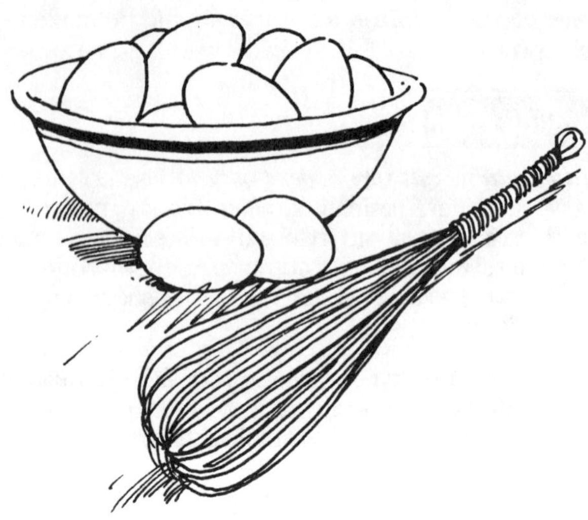

Eggs: A Major Contributor of Cholesterol to the American Diet

You Need Eggs-Pertise!

The cholesterol controversy lingers on. It appears that what is important to most of us is to reduce the total fat in the diet, especially saturated fats. However, for individuals with an elevated blood cholesterol level, it is important to reduce dietary cholesterol as well as total fat. Foods high in dietary cholesterol are eggs, liver and other organ meats.

It is recommended that you limit your use of egg yolk to no more than three per week, and your total dietary cholesterol to less than 300 milligrams per day. A single large egg contains between 250 to 275 milligrams of cholesterol concentrated totally in the yolk, nearly your entire day's quota of cholesterol. The bulk of calories (90 calories per large egg) are also contained in the egg yolk.

Egg whites, on the other hand, are an excellent low-calorie source of protein. By separating out whites from yolks, this protein source can still be a very versatile food item in your kitchen. Contrary to popular belief, raw eggs provide no extra nutritional boost for athletes in training or for improving hair, skin or toenails. Actually, cooking eggs increases the availability of the B vitamin biotin and destroys any food poisoning bacteria that may be present in raw eggs.

Egg substitutes may be a valuable dietary aid for those with elevated blood cholesterol. (They were developed for use by individuals trying to lower cholesterol, much in the same way artificially sweetened jams were developed for people with diabetes.) These substitutes are egg white preparations with added starch, nonfat dry milk and vitamin enrichment. They are available in powder and liquid forms. Depending on the brand you choose, they may be lower in calories as well as cholesterol.

Shopping Tips

- The color of an egg shell or of the egg yolk makes no difference in the nutritional quality of the egg. The color is determined by the variety of chicken from which the egg came, and white or brown makes no difference.

Cooking Tips

- To make your own egg substitute, use the following proportions:

  1 dozen large egg whites
  1 egg yolk
  1/2 cup nonfat dry milk
  1/2 tsp. yellow food coloring

  Mix well. You can use it in any way you would use beaten eggs. One-half cup equals two eggs, and contains 56 calories and 14 grams of protein.

- Decreasing your daily intake of cholesterol need not mean you use only egg substitutes. When preparing eggs for a meal, simply discard every other yolk. For example, make your omelet with two egg whites and one yolk. You can do the same with pancakes and French toast without sacrificing taste.

- Use two egg whites for one whole egg or three egg whites for two eggs. Adding a teaspoon of salad oil will help to replace the missing yolk's nonstick properties.

- Separate eggs when they are cold. The yolk is firmest in a chilled egg, and there is less chance of it running into the white portion.

- Egg whites whip better at room temperature, so after the eggs have been separated, you'll get more volume if you let them warm up a bit.

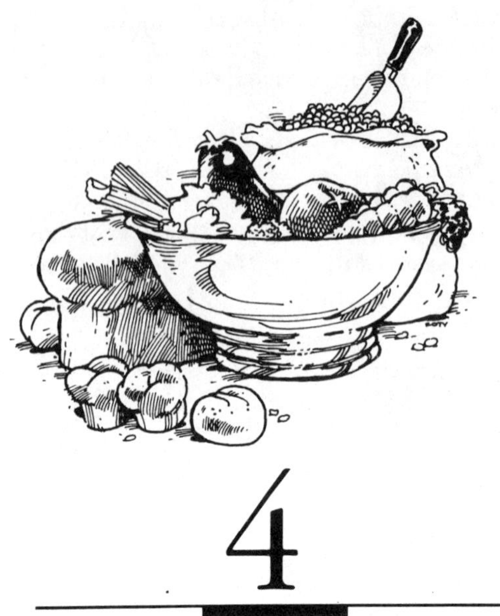

4

TEAM UP WITH CARBOHYDRATES TO INCREASE DIETARY FIBER

The next key to opening the door to a nutritious and healthy lifestyle is to eat more complex carbohydrates, fiber and "naturally occurring" sugars. We'll explain each in turn.

Dietary carbohydrate should be primarily from vegetables, fruits, and whole grain enriched breads and cereals, making up about 50 to 60 percent of your calories. Fruits, vegetables and grains are important sources of calories and nutrients. All add variety, are highly versatile, economical, and easy to prepare. In addition, they are cholesterol free and low in fat. For these reasons, their use is encouraged.

Ounce for ounce, starches contain the same number of calories as pure protein and less than half the calories of fat. As an example, one slice of bread or a medium potato contains approximately 70 to 80 calories. One ounce of a medium to high fat meat contains 80 to 100 calories!

Many people erroneously believe that carbohydrate foods are

fattening. But what can make carbohydrate foods fattening are the high-calorie sauces, creams, dressings and fats often added to these foods. And remember, all food is fattening when consumed in excess.

Complex carbohydrates are starches found in breads, cereals, starchy vegetables, legumes and pastas. A good source of vitamins, minerals and fiber, complex carbohydrates can also help control weight if they are used to replace fats and refined carbohydrates in the diet. These foods have considerably fewer calories than do foods with high fat or sugar content.

"Naturally occurring" sugars are found in fruits, milk and milk products, and vegetables. These foods also contain significant amounts of vitamins and minerals. Refined and processed sugars are found in candy, syrups, honey, molasses, regular soda pops, etc. These foods provide calories but few or no nutrients.

Fiber is a component of food that is resistant to being digested or absorbed by the small intestine. Fiber has been shown to lower blood cholesterol and triglyceride levels and to reduce the symptoms of chronic constipation and diverticulosis (formation of pockets in the intestine). Fiber also satisfies the need for bulk in the diet and leaves you feeling "full."

Whole grain cereals and breads, raw vegetables and fruits with edible skins are important sources of fiber. Unprocessed wheat bran is one of the richest sources of fiber. Nuts and seeds provide a certain amount of fiber as well. The fiber in cereals and grains is not the same as the fiber found in fruits and vegetables. Different types of fiber serve different functions. To get a full variety of fiber, eat a variety of plant foods with fiber: fruits, vegetables, cereals, legumes, seeds and nuts.

TYPES OF FIBER AND SIGNIFICANT FOOD SOURCES

Type	Source
Hemicellulose and cellulose	Legumes, nuts, grains, vegetables, fruits, bran
Pectin	Fruits
Gum and Mucilage	Beans, seeds
Lignin	Vegetables, beans

Fiber can also be divided according to solubility (ability to dissolve) in water. Fiber from fruits (pectin), legumes (gum), and oats are water soluble. Water soluble fibers form a gel during digestion and thus are absorbed slower. These fibers then may be helpful in lowering blood sugar. Oat bran and dried beans (pinto, navy, kidney, etc.) have the added advantage of lowering your blood cholesterol levels. Fibers from grains and wheat bran are water insoluble. They reduce the time it takes food to pass through the intestine and are useful if constipation is a problem.

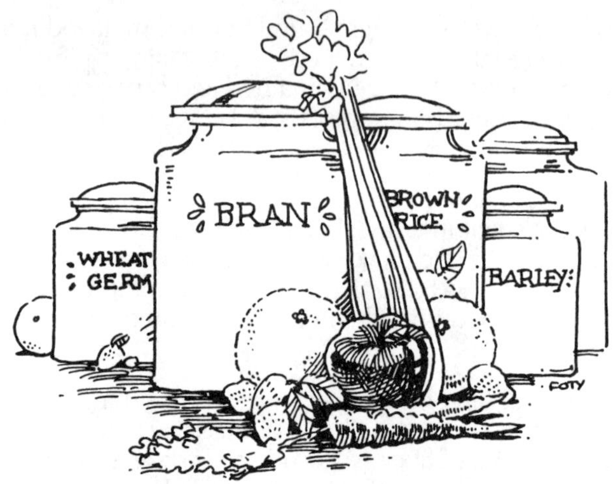

The following food groups are excellent sources of fiber:

- ***Fruits*** — Select fruits with edible skins and seeds. They can be fresh, frozen, canned or dried. Eat more whole fruits in place of fruit juices. One serving (1/2 cup or one medium fruit) has an average of 2 grams of fiber and 40 to 60 calories (1 fruit exchange).

- ***Vegetables*** — Choose vegetables with edible skins and seeds. These too may be fresh, frozen or canned. One to two cups raw or 1/2 to 3/4 cup cooked vegetables has an average of 2 grams of fiber and 25 calories (1 vegetable exchange).

- ***Starchy Vegetables*** — These are slightly higher in calories than other vegetables but still an excellent source of fiber and bulk. One serving averages 3 grams of fiber and 70 calories (1 bread exchange). Good choices in this category are:

Starchy Foods	Average Serving Size
Barley, cooked	1/2 cup
Corn, cooked	1/2 cup
Cracked wheat (bulgur)	1/4 cup
Green peas, cooked	1/2 cup
Parsnips, cooked	3/4 cup
Potatoes, baked with skin	1 small
Rice, brown or wild, cooked	1/3 cup
Squash, winter	1/2 cup
Sweet potatoes, cooked	1/4 cup

- ***Breads, Grains and Cereals*** — Choose breads, cereals and crackers made from grains that retain their natural fibrous coatings. For whole grain breads, look for whole grain, whole wheat, cracked wheat, stone ground, whole meal or rye flour as the first or second item on the ingredient list. (Wheat flour on an ingredient list is usually white flour.) One serving of bread or grains averages 2 grams of fiber and 70 calories (1 bread exchange). Good choices in this category are:

Bread and Bread Products	Average Serving Size
Graham crackers	2 squares
*Millers unprocessed bran	1 Tbsp.
Muffins: bran, oat, corn	½ muffin
Popcorn	3 cups
Rye crackers (Rye Krisp)	3 squares
Rye, pumpernickel, whole wheat or whole meal bread	1 slice
Whole wheat crackers	6
Whole wheat rolls	1

*1.5 grams fiber and 0 calories

One serving of cereal averages 3 grams of fiber and 70 calories. The table on the next page shows good choices.

Cereal	Average Serving Size
*All Bran or 100% Bran	1/2 cup
*Bran Buds	1/3 cup
Bran Chex	1/2 cup
Bran Flakes (40% bran)	3/4 cup
Bran Flakes with Raisins	1/3 cup
Corn Bran	1/2 cup
Corn Chex	3/4 cup
Corn Flakes	3/4 cup
Grapenuts	1/4 cup
Grapenut Flakes	2/3 cup
Grits	1/4 cup
**Nutri Grains	1/2 cup
†Oat Bran	1/4 cup
Oatmeal	1/2 cup
Post Toasties	1 cup
Puffed Wheat	1¼ cup
Ralstons or rolled whole wheat, cooked	1/2 cup
Rolled whole oats, cooked (oatmeal)	1/2 cup
Shredded Wheat	1 biscuit
Total	3/4 cup
Wheaties	3/4 cup

*8 grams fiber
**2 grams fiber
†5 grams fiber

- ***Legumes, Nuts and Seeds*** — Fiber is found in cooked or canned dried beans (lima, kidney, navy, pinto, etc.), dried peas and lentils. All varieties of nuts as well as pumpkin, sesame and sunflower seeds contain fiber. One-half cup cooked beans, peas or lentils averages 8 grams of fiber and 90 calories (1 bread exchange). One ounce of nuts or seeds has an average of 3 grams of fiber and 190 calories (1 medium meat and 2 fat exchanges).

There are several things you can do to increase fiber intake: Eat more raw or slightly cooked vegetables. Use fruits rather than fruit juices. Whenever possible, do not peel them. Choose whole grain breads, cereals, crackers and pastas, and gradually substitute whole grains for more refined foods. Dried peas, beans and legumes are also excellent sources of fiber.

Add fiber gradually to your diet. If fiber is added too rapidly, some people complain of feeling "stuffed," "bloated," and "gassy." Also, drink extra fluids to prevent fiber from causing constipation.

Reduce Intake of Refined Sugar.
How Naturally Sweet It Is!

The recommendation to increase complex carbohydrates (starches) and "naturally occurring" sugars implies a decreased consumption of refined or concentrated sweets. Sweets contain simple sugars such as sucrose, dextrose and honey. Sweets can contribute a large amount of calories without any important nutrients; therefore, these calories are known as "empty" calories. Frequently sweet foods are high in fat as well.

There is currently no evidence to indicate that sugar intake is a risk factor in any particular disease, except perhaps dental caries (cavities). A moderate amount of sweets in the diet will not be a problem, and indeed small amounts can contribute to the enjoyment of eating.

The occurrence of tooth decay depends not only on the amount of sugar eaten but also on the frequency and degree of stickiness of the sugar food. Tooth decay is caused because bacteria which live in the mouth use sugar as food for growth. The bacteria produce weak acids that can dissolve tooth enamel. Foods that contain sticky forms of sugar, such as taffy-like candies and sugar-coated cereals, are the most likely to cause tooth decay, especially when eaten between meals.

Although humans have no inborn salt craving or urge for fat, we naturally like sweetness. Animals too, with the exception of cats, have a "sweet tooth." However, many humans have fed their "sweet tooth" so well that they crave unhealthy levels of sugar.

Most of the sugar we eat comes concealed in the form of food products and beverages such as soft drinks, candy, pastries, donuts, cakes, cookies, sugared cereals, ice cream and other sweet desserts, as well as from jams, jellies, table sugar, honey, molasses and fructose. The soda pop industry is the major user of sugar today—a 12-ounce can of soda pop contains 8 to 10 teaspoons of sugar.

The key is to reduce your intake of refined (table sugar) and processed sugars (used in baked goods or in the manufacturing process of many other foods.) These sugars currently contribute 25 percent of the average American's total calories, or the equivalent of 12 tablespoons of sugar daily. An appropriate goal is to reduce sugar to approximately 10 percent of the total energy intake.

The following gives you some idea of foods that contain sugar:

SNACKS AND DESSERTS:	SUGAR (teaspoons)
Marshmallows (2 average)	3
Cookies (2 medium)	3
Brownie (2″ × 2″ × 3/4″)	3
Fruits canned in heavy syrup	3
Ice cream (1 cup)	6
Chocolate cake with icing (1 slice)	7-8
Chocolate sauce (2 Tbsp.)	7-8
Poptarts (one)	3-4
Doughnut, plain (1 medium)	3-4
Apple Pie (1 slice)	3-4
Popsicle	4.5
Fruit-flavored yogurt (8 oz.)	6-7.5
Twinkie (1 pkg.)	8.4

BEVERAGES:	SUGAR (teaspoons)
Kool-aid sugar sweetened (8 oz.)	5-6
Chocolate milkshake, "Fast Food" (10 oz.)	5
Hawaiian Punch (8 oz.)	6.5
Ginger Ale (12 oz.)	8
Dry Tonic Water (12 oz.)	8.4
Sprite (12 oz.)	9-10
Coca-Cola (12 oz.)	9-10
Seven-up (12 oz.)	9-10

SWEETENERS:	SUGAR (teaspoons)
Maple syrup (¼ cup, average serving)	8
Pancake and waffle syrup (¼ cup)	14

CANDY:	SUGAR (teaspoons)
Jelly beans (10 pieces)	6.6
M & M's (1.7 oz.)	4.8-6.6
Candy bars (2 oz.)	7-9
"Slender Bars" (2 oz.)	4-4.8

To Reduce Refined and Processed Sugars:

- To satisfy your "sweet tooth," eat fruits, low-fat dairy products or breads with ingredients such as oatmeal, whole wheat flour, raisins, nuts, pumpkin, zucchini, carrots or peanut butter instead of eating cakes, cookies, or pies.
- Honey, raw sugar, brown sugar and other so-called "natural sweeteners" are no more nourishing than refined sugar. Their mineral content is so low that you would have to consume all your day's calories in sugar just to get a significant amount of vitamins and minerals. These sugars, like refined sugar, provide only sweetness and calories.
- Honey contains fructose, a sweetener that is digested differently than table sugar. However, these differences have little actual effect. Fructose, like table sugar, ends up as glucose, the food substance your body needs for energy. After absorption of glucose from the intestine, the body does not know if the glucose came from honey, table sugar or some other carbohydrate. The advantage of many of the starches and "naturally occurring" sugars is that each carries essential vitamins and minerals along with the glucose.
- Avoid buying sweet snacks to have in the house. Cut back on commercial baked goods such as pastries, sweet rolls and cookies, which are the second biggest source of sugar after soft drinks.
- Dessert powders such as Jello are 85 percent sugar and 10 percent gelatin plus factory-made flavoring and color.
- One candy bar has as much sugar as 1/2 pound of apples.
- An average serving of pancake syrup is 1/4 cup. This is as much sugar as four to five apples or oranges.
- Substitute fruit juices, skim milk and water for soft drinks.
- Calories per 12 ounces of soft drinks (primarily from sugar):

Fruit flavored pops	170
Root Beer	150
Cola	145
Ginger Ale	115
Quinine Sodas	115
Lo Cal Sodas	0-2
Club Soda	0

The soft drink industry is the largest single source of sugar in the diet. The sugar in one 12-ounce can of cola supplies 145 calories—calories unaccompanied by other nutrients.

Along with carbonated water and sugar, (either sucrose, dextrose, fructose or high fructose syrup) other typical ingredients in soft drinks include caramel coloring, phosphoric acid and possibly citric acid, caffeine, and the flavoring used in the secret formulas. Most caffeinated colas contain between 35 and 50 milligrams of caffeine per 12-ounce can, or about the amount in one-third of a cup of strong brewed coffee.

Diet soft drinks continue to be very popular even though there is no convincing evidence that they help in the control or loss of weight. One theory is that people who drink diet soda feel it allows them to eat extra cake, cookies and candy.

Diet sodas currently account for about 20 percent of the soft drink market, which translates into something like 20 billion cans of diet soda a year, much of it consumed by women.

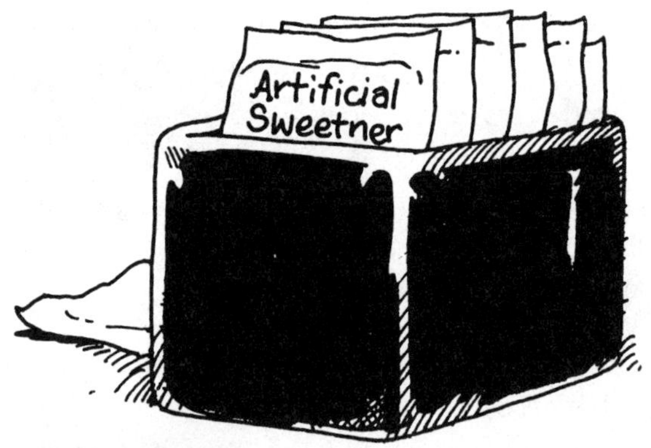

Shopping Tips

- Check ingredient labels on packages for clues to the sugar content. If sugar appears first, the product is relatively high in sugar. If the label lists sucrose, dextrose, glucose, lactose, fructose, maltose, galactose, corn syrup, invert sugar, honey, molasses or maple syrup, you should check to see how many of these ingredients are in the product, because all are forms of sugar.
- Adding water may reduce the percentage of sugar without actually changing the amount in the product. Percentages can be misleading. As an example, a glass of cola has a lower percentage of sugar than a bouillon cube but actually contains significantly more

sugar. It is more helpful to know the actual number of grams of sugar contained in the product.

- Metric measurements are still unfamiliar to many people, and can be confusing when used on products. The 11 grams of sugar in a one-ounce serving of frosted flakes is the same as adding one tablespoon of sugar to your bowl of cereal.
- The words "dietetic" or "sugar free" do not always mean a product is low in calories or carbohydrate. The ingredients most often used to sweeten "dietetic" products are sorbitol and mannitol, which are carbohydrates just like sugar. In fact, most of these so-called "dietetic" products are higher in calories than the regular products because of added fat.

CALORIC CONTENT OF DIETETIC SWEETS

Dietetic Product	Calories	Regular Product	Calories
½ cup "dietetic" ice cream	180	½ cup regular ice cream	140
1 chocolate chip "dietetic" cookie 1¾″ in diameter	41	1 chocolate chip cookie, 1¾″ in diameter	36
1 3-oz. "dietetic" chocolate candy bar	535	1 3-oz. chocolate candy bar	320

Cooking Tips

- Sugar and other sweeteners add flavor, color, tenderness and crispness in baked products. In many recipes, you can reduce the amount of sugar called for by at least 1/3 to 1/2 without affecting the quality of the product. A helpful guideline: use no more than 1/4 cup of added sweetener (sugar, honey, molasses, etc.) per one cup of flour. Every 1/4 cup of sugar adds close to 200 empty calories to your recipes.
- Adding extra vanilla will enhance the sweetness of a recipe. Vanilla, cinnamon and nutmeg all give the illusion of sweetness without adding calories.
- Select fresh fruits or fruits canned without sugar instead of fruits canned in heavy syrup.

- Learn to sweeten with naturally occurring sugars, such as undiluted fruit juice concentrate. Several tablespoons of thawed apple juice concentrate can often be substituted for refined sugar to provide the necessary sweetness. Of course, the apple juice is sweet, but naturally—from fructose. It has 30 calories in one tablespoon compared to 45 in a tablespoon of sugar. And you will probably not need to use as much apple juice as you would sugar. Orange juice can also be used.

  You will need to experiment to discover in which recipes substitutions can be made. Baked foods, especially cakes, cookies and breads, require some sugar, although the amount can usually be reduced. Use the juice for sweetening other fruit beverages, fruit gelatins, yogurt, puddings, sour fruits, fruit toppings and some desserts. If you do start experimenting with fruit juices in place of sugar, decrease the liquid in the original recipe by about the same amount as the added juice.

- In place of syrup, the following excellent topping can be used:
  Ingredients—2 cups fresh or frozen-without-sugar blueberries, strawberries or other fruit
  2 teaspoons undiluted frozen apple juice concentrate

  Directions—Combine 1/2 cup of the fruit and 2 teaspoons apple juice concentrate in a blender and process to a smooth sauce. Pour this over the remaining fruit. It will make four half-cup servings. Top with a dollop of plain yogurt and serve on waffles, pancakes, etc. One-half cup equals 40 to 60 calories (10 grams of carbohydrate or one fruit exchange). An average serving of regular syrup, 1/4 cup, has 60 grams of carbohydrate and 240 calories. (From *Cooking to Stay in SHAPE.)*

- ***Equal®*** is a tabletop sweetener that has a taste similar to sugar with only 1/8 the calories. Since it does not contain saccharin, it does not have a synthetic flavor or a bitter, metallic aftertaste. Equal contains the ***NutraSweet™*** brand of aspartame, which is a combination of two amino acids (the building blocks of protein)—aspartic acid and phenylalanine. Aspartame achieves the same sweetness as sugar with only 1/200th the calories. It is broken down in the body like protein, but it can be harmful to people with a rare inherited metabolic abnormality called phenylketonuria or PKU. A warning to people with PKU appears on packages of Equal and products sweetened with NutraSweet. Equal is available in single serving packets and tablets. One packet is as sweet as 2 teaspoons of sugar (32 calories) but supplies only 4 calories. Each tablet is as sweet as one teaspoon of sugar but contributes only 1/4 the calories.

Equal can be used to sweeten foods and beverages in which you would normally use table sugar. Use it in simple recipes that do not require heating, because Equal loses sweetness when exposed to heat. In addition, Equal does not provide the necessary bulk and structure required in home-baked foods such as cakes, breads and cookies.

The high heat needed for home canning will cause Equal to lose its sweetness, but jams, jellies, fruit butters and other preserves can be made with it for freezer storage.

- ***When using Equal, remember the following:***
  Allow cooked fruits to cool before sweetening with Equal. Mousses, puddings, gelatins and other chilled desserts can be made with Equal, as can ice cream, sherbet and other frozen desserts. For fresh fruits, cereals, coffee, tea or unsweetened fruit drinks, add Equal directly.

Questions concerning the safety of aspartame have been raised. Aspartame underwent more than 100 scientific studies to establish its safety. Various safety concerns raised during the 16 years of aspartame's development and approval were addressed by the FDA. In each case, FDA concluded that the various safety concerns raised were not supported by scientific evidence.

One of the issues raised is that in the body, aspartame breaks down rapidly into methanol, which the critics said is harmful to the person consuming it. To understand why this is not so, consider: If the average daily amount of sugar consumed by a person in the United States were replaced by aspartame (which would be virtually impossible to do, because sugar is our leading food additive), it would produce 280 milligrams of phenylalanine, 226 milligrams of aspartic acid, and 54 milligrams of methanol. These amounts of phenylalanine and aspartic acid are less than the quantities provided by 6 ounces of milk or 3 ounces of beef. The same amount of methanol is provided by 8 ounces of fruit or vegetable juice or 2 ounces of gin. As you can see, many foods such as fruit, fruit juices, tomato juice, vegetable soup, and alcohol all break down into methanol. The methanol from the breakdown of aspartame is the same as the methanol produced in the human body from food.

Another issue raised is that phenylalanine, one of the two primary components of aspartame, can cause changes in the brain's chemistry and result in behavioral changes, particularly in children. At expected levels of intake, phenylalanine levels do not exceed those observed after normal meals. Even at abusive intake levels, the amount of phenylalanine in the blood is below amounts expected to show toxic effects. A panel convened by the FDA concluded that the evidence did not support the charge that aspartame might harm the brain, but they did recommend that long-term animal studies be conducted.

The FDA has concluded that an acceptable daily intake of aspartame is up to 50 milligrams per kilogram (2.2 pounds) of body weight. If all sugar in the average person's diet were replaced with aspartame the resulting intake would be 34 milligrams per kilogram. A 12-ounce can of diet soda contains approximately 150-200 milligrams of aspartame, which is less than 3 milligrams per kilogram for a 150-pound person.

Studies have found no evidence of adverse effects even at levels of aspartame consumption six times greater than what 99 percent of the general public could be expected to consume. Dr. David Horwitz of the Department of Medicine, University of Illinois Medical Center, has concluded that "aspartame thus appears to meet our expectations for a safe, low-calorie sweetener with no undesirable after-taste."

To Increase Complex Carbohydrates and Fiber While Reducing Refined Sugar:

1. Increase use of fruits and vegetables.
2. Increase use of grains and rice, flours and breads.
3. Increase use of legumes (e.g. beans, peas and lentils).
4. Choose whole grain cereals.
5. Choose "natural-occurring" sugars as much as possible for desserts.

Fruits

Fresh fruits are excellent choices for the health conscious. Besides adding a sweet, nutritious flair to any meal, they are excellent sources of "naturally occurring" sugar. Fruits also provide important vitamins and minerals, especially vitamins A and C.

FRUITS HIGH IN VITAMIN C		FRUITS HIGH IN VITAMIN A	
Cantaloupe	Oranges	Apricots	Persimmon
Grapefruit	Papaya	Cantaloupe	Nectarines
Honeydew Melon	Red Raspberries	Grapefruit	Mangos
Lemons	Strawberries	Ground Cherries	
Mangos	Tangerines		

Ascorbic acid (vitamin C) has been shown to enhance iron absorption from other foods eaten at the same meal. However, the vitamin C must be taken during the meal for the increased iron absorption effect to take place. Citrus fruits are excellent sources of vitamin C.

Dried fruits make excellent snacks and are a great substitute for candy. Iron, a mineral that is lacking in most diets, can be obtained while enjoying many of the dried fruits.

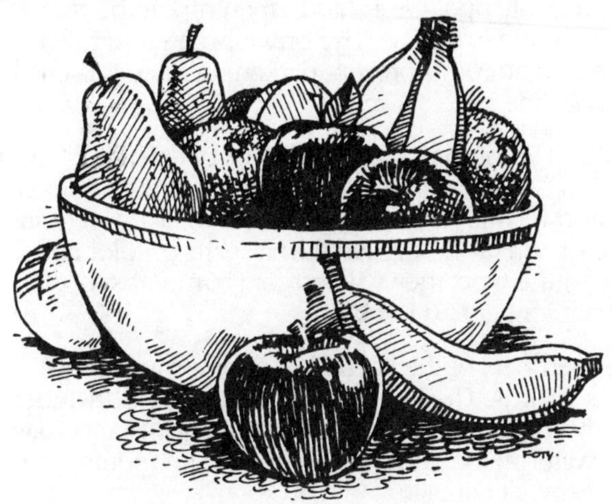

To increase fiber in your diet, select fruits with edible skins or seeds. Fruits high in fiber are apricots, apples, avocados, bananas, berries, coconut, dates, figs, grapes, grapefruit, oranges, peaches, pears, prunes, raisins, rhubarb and tangerines. These can be fresh, frozen, canned or dried.

The American Dental Association has emphasized the importance of choosing fruits such as apples and oranges or uncooked vegetables such as carrots and celery as the last food eaten at a meal or snack. Such "detergent foods" cleanse the teeth and soft tissues of food debris, helping to prevent tooth decay.

Now that we've looked at the uses and value of fruit, let's discuss some specific members of this food family.

Apricots, a significant source of potassium, are an especially good source of iron as well. Two fresh apricots contain only 36 calories. Apricots can be added to recipes for a natural sweet flavor in place of syrup, sugar or honey. When pureed or mashed, apricots become thick and creamy and are a good substitute for fats and cream in many recipes.

Avocados, unlike most fruits that are high in carbohydrates, contain as much as 17 percent oil (by total weight of edible fruit). The fat content provides 76 to 89 percent of their total calories, which is why they are usually included on fat lists. However, the fat is a monounsaturated oil.

The best avocados are generally free of bruises, but irregular markings known as "scabs" are only superficial and do not affect the flavor or flesh. To test for ripeness, cradle the fruit in the hand. If it is soft to the touch, it is probably ripe. If it is hard, ripening can be hurried by placing the avocado in a paper bag or wrapping it in foil and leaving it at room temperature. To prevent darkening once it is cut, brush it with lemon or lime juice.

Dates are about 73 percent sugar and have been called "candy that grows on trees." Along with this naturally sweet taste comes a small amount of iron (1 milligram per 100 calories). Dates require a temperature of 32 F to best retain flavor, texture, color and aroma. Depending on the type, they will last for six months to a year at 32 F and somewhat longer at 0 F.

Melons are members of the cucumber family. Melons may otherwise be known as gourds. The varieties of sweet melons include cantaloupe, honeydew, casaba, crenshaw, Persian, Santa Claus (or Christmas), watermelon and canary. All of them require careful handling to prevent damage.

The sweetness and flavor of melons does not completely develop until a full-ripe stage of maturity is reached. Total sugar content does not increase once the melon is cut from the vine, so an immature melon will not ripen. Ripeness is indicated by the softening of the fruit surrounding the "eye" or "button" at the blossom end, which yields to gentle pressure of the finger. Most melons have an odor which becomes stronger when they have fully ripened.

Nectarines and peaches do not gain sugar once they have been picked, so they must be harvested at maturity. Holding them at room temperature for two to three days is usually enough to complete ripening. To select a nectarine, look for a creamy yellow background and well-formed fruit without bruises. The crimson blush of nectarines is an indication of variety, not maturity. A bright, fresh appearance is a good clue to a high-quality peach, while a greenish color suggests that the peach was immature when picked and will not ripen well. Such a peach will become shriveled or flabby and have tough or poorly flavored skin. A red blush is an indication of the variety, not a true sign of quality.

Pears, unlike other fruit, are harvested while the skin is still green and the flesh is firm, because they won't ripen properly on the tree. Fruit that is allowed to ripen on the tree will develop a coarse, woody or gritty texture. Green pears will ripen for eating by putting them in a loosely closed bag. Keep them together, because pears give off gases that aid each other in ripening.

Prunes are especially known for their high iron and potassium contents. They contain a natural laxative—not yet completely identified chemically—which acts as a regulator of the large intestine. Prunes keep best when stored in a cool, dry place. For long-term storage, keep them in the refrigerator.

Shopping Tips

- One week is the maximum storage time for nearly all fresh fruits, except apples and citrus fruits. As a rule, don't buy fresh fruits in large amounts or keep them for any great length of time.
- Many fresh fruits are ready to use when purchased: apples, cherries, citrus fruits, berries, grapes and pineapples. Others require additional ripening to bring out maximum flavor. These include avocados, bananas, melons, mangos, peaches, plums, pears, nectarines and papayas. They can be held at room temperature until they reach the desired degree of ripeness, then they can be refrigerated a few days. To hasten the ripening process, keep fruit in a brown bag at room temperature, checking daily.
- When purchasing canned fruit, choose those packed in water or their own fruit juice. When purchasing frozen fruit, choose those that have been frozen plain, with no sugar added.
- If the label says "fruit drink," "ade," "nectar" or "punch," beware. A "juice drink" is only 50 percent juice, "ade" is 20 percent juice and a "drink" is only 10 percent juice. No mandatory amount of juice is set for "nectar" or "punch," but all contain sugar, water, artificial color and flavor. If a fruit "juice" has sugar added, it must be stated on the label. Juices do not need to be labeled "unsweetened" or "no sugar added."

Cooking Tips

- Wash fresh fruits thoroughly just before serving them raw or cooked. Carefully rinse fresh berries before using.

- To peel plums, nectarines and peaches easily, submerge them in boiling water for 30 seconds, remove with a slotted spoon and dip in cold water. The skins will slip off easily.
- To prevent apples, pears, peaches and bananas from discoloring when cut or peeled, dip them into citrus fruit juices (lemon, lime, orange or grapefruit).
- To preserve nutrients when cooking fresh fruits and vegetables, reduce the amount of water and cooking time and minimize the amount of surface area exposed to air by doing as little cutting, paring and shredding as possible.
- Fruits for desserts can be whole (baked or poached), sliced (sauteed, flambeed, fresh in salad), pureed (in toppings and beverages), dried (stewed with spirits, juices or extracts), canned or frozen (in salads or alone).

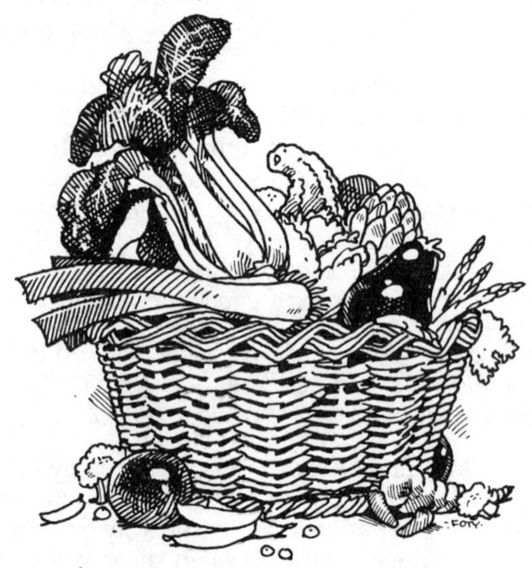

Vegetables

Many factors control the nutritive value of vegetables, among them climate, season of harvesting, soil, storage and preparation. Despite those variables, some generalizations can be made. Seed vegetables, such as peas and beans, are good sources of vitamin B (thiamine) and a fair source of riboflavin. They are among the best vegetable sources of protein and iron. Green leaves are an important source of riboflavin, vitamin C and iron. Leafy green vegetables offer significant amounts of calcium as well.

Vegetables high in dietary fiber are: asparagus, beets, bean sprouts, broccoli, Brussels sprouts, cabbage, carrots, cauliflower, corn, eggplant, green beans, green peas, green pepper, leafy greens, lima beans, potatoes, rutabagas, squash and sweet potatoes.

A real bonus to calorie counters is that an average 1/2-cup serving of most vegetables is between 25 and 50 calories. A serving of the more starchy varieties, such as lima beans, peas, corn and boiled potatoes, is between 50 and 100 calories.

Shopping Tips

- When fresh vegetables are not available, your best alternative is frozen vegetables. Frozen foods have their highest overall nutritional quality if consumed within their shelf-life period. Industrial methods of quick freezing also minimize nutrient losses and retard microorganism growth.

  These advantages can be greatly diminished, however, depending on the method you use to thaw your frozen products. Rapid thawing, like rapid freezing, maintains the highest food quality by decreasing nutrient losses and the possibility of bacterial growth and food poisoning.

  Thawing at room temperature is the least recommended method, because of the chance of microorganism growth while the food sits out on the counter top. Instead, use boil-in-the-bag vegetables (look for those varieties that aren't in heavy butter sauces), cook right from the frozen state, or thaw and cook in a microwave.

- Whenever possible, purchase fresh or frozen vegetables rather than canned. Many vitamins will dissolve into the water used in canning or be destroyed by the high temperatures involved. Canned vegetables are also processed with large amounts of salt.

- Most carrots are sold without tops, which have been shown to withdraw moisture from the roots. Carrots without tops also store better. Watch for color: carrots with large green areas at the top are undesirable, while a darker orange color indicates more vitamin A. Carrots retain their vitamin A content well in storage.

- Spinach can be stored for three to five days if refrigerated. Spinach that is straggly, long-stemmed or overgrown with seed stalks will be undesirable, as will plants with coarse leaf stems that may be tough.

- Tomato quality is mostly dependent on proper harvesting and handling methods. If a tomato is picked mature when still green, it will ship well and ripen to a good flavor and quality. If it is picked immature, flavor and coloring will suffer.

  Most fresh tomatoes sold in supermarkets are firm and not yet ripe. To hasten ripening, place fresh tomatoes in a brown paper bag. As the fruit ripens, it emits a natural gas called ethylene. This gas speeds up the ripening process when confined around the fruit in a closed bag. Allow the tomatoes to ripen at room temperature, away from direct sunlight. Fresh tomatoes should not be refrigerated before they are fully ripe—cold temperatures will diminish the flavor, texture and aroma.

  Ripe tomatoes should be completely red or reddish-orange and give slightly to gentle pressure. Once tomatoes have ripened, they may be kept in the refrigerator for several days.

- Shop often for fresh vegetables and choose produce that has been ripened on the vine whenever possible. This will minimize vitamin losses due to storage.

- When purchasing canned vegetables, read the ingredients list and avoid products with added sugar and many sources of sodium.

Cooking Tips

- Vegetables add color, crispness and deep, rich flavor to any menu. However, be careful of adding glazes, butter, margarine or sauces to vegetables. These add unnecessary fats and calories.

- Varieties of salad greens are: iceberg, Boston, Bibb, leaf (romaine), spinach, endive, chicory and escarole. A crisp leaf (romaine) can accomodate a stronger dressing than a more delicate leaf (Boston). When cleaning greens, remove all dirt from the surface of the leaf. If the salad is to be made immediately, the greens should be thoroughly dried. This keeps them crisp and helps dressing cling to the surface. If the greens will be used later, they can be wrapped in a damp paper towel and placed in the refrigerator. But be careful—if the towel is too wet, greens may rot.

- Vegetables should be stored at appropriate temperature. If temperatures are too cold, the cells are robbed of needed moisture. If too warm, they will wilt. Don't overexpose vegetables to light.

- To preserve water-soluble vitamins (B and C), avoid prolonged soaking of fresh vegetables. Also delay cutting and cooking vegetables until the last minute.

- For recipes that call for vegetables to be sauteed in oil, try sauteeing in a small amount of broth instead. This will reduce fat in the recipe and add flavor as well. Or the vegetables can be cooked in a microwave oven for a few minutes. Reduce the salt called for in the recipe as well.

- Probably the most important thing when cooking vegetables is not to overcook them. The amount of tenderness you desire is a matter of personal taste, but nutritionally there is no such thing as an undercooked vegetable.

- Steaming vegetables is a good way to preserve their nutritional value. When steaming broccoli or other dark green vegetables, leave the lid slightly ajar to allow the steam to escape in order to preserve the nice green color. This allows volatile acids to escape which would otherwise cause vegetables to turn gray-green. Any overcooked vegetables will turn color, however.

- Cook your favorite vegetable in as little time—and liquid—as possible. Try simmering vegetables in a self-making sauce based on unsweetened fruit juice and cornstarch. Three-fourths pound fresh vegetables simmered in 3/4 cup unsweetened juice with 1/2 teaspoon cornstarch creates a delightful, slightly sweet glaze at only 45 calories per 1/2 cup serving.

- Freeze cooked vegetables for soups, stews and casseroles. For a great salad, chill and combine drained leftover vegetables with seasonings and salad dressing.

- The addition of herbs and spices enhances the flavor of vegetables and can be used in place of butter on vegetables. Try the following:

  Basil with tomatoes.
  Chopped chives and parsley, sprinkled on just before serving, enhance the flavor of many vegetables.
  Marjoram with Brussels sprouts, carrots or spinach.
  Oregano with zucchini, Brussels sprouts, carrots, and spinach.
  Rosemary with peas, cauliflower and spinach.

- To fix baked potatoes that don't require any added butter or sour cream, try the following idea from ***Cooking to Stay in SHAPE***: Cut the potato in half. Brush each half with melted margarine and sprinkle with paprika and Parmesan cheese. Then place them skin up on an oiled cookie sheet and bake at 350 degrees for 25 to 30 minutes or until the potato is fork tender. Each half will contain 84 calories and 1 gram of fat. (For people on an exchange meal plan, 1/2 large potato equals 1 bread exchange.)

- ***Hungry for French fries?*** Try fresh sliced potatoes tossed with a small amount of oil and oven baked at 450 to 500 until brown.

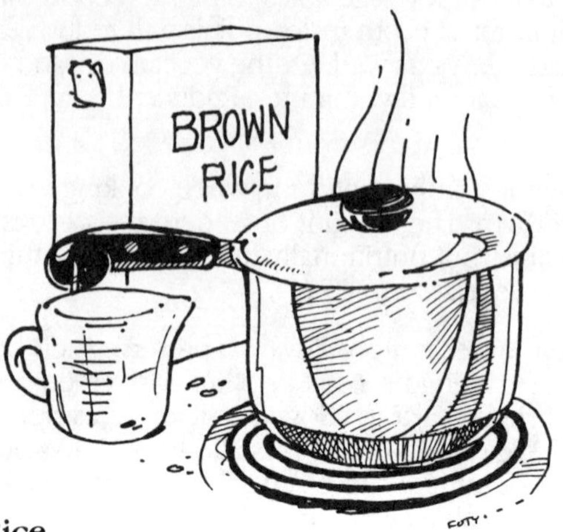

Grains and Rice

Grain products supply protein, B vitamins, iron and energy. An average slice of bread contains approximately 70 calories. Adding a tablespoon of honey, preserves or butter doubles the calories!

Whole grains such as barley, bran, brown rice, buckwheat grouts (kasha), bulgur (cracked wheat), cornmeal, popcorn, whole wheat and wheat germ provide excellent sources of fiber in the diet.

Shopping Tips

The grain group consists of barley, corn, oats, rice, rye, wheat (bulgur, wheatgerm, sprouts), as well as flours and cereals made from these grains. Try experimenting with a variety of grains.

- *Barley* — Although the outer hull has been removed from barley, the kernel still contains the endosperm that is mostly protein, the bean that contains B vitamins, and the germ or sprouting section that contains fiber, making barley a nutritious food. The cooked barley kernels have a nut-like flavor with a slightly chewy texture.

  When you shop for barley, remember that there are two types: pearled regular and pearled quick barley. "Pearled" means that the outer hull has been removed and polished. Regular pearled barley, a common ingredient in soups and stews, takes about an hour to cook. The quick pearled barley, because of special processing, takes only about 10 minutes cooking time.

  The uses for barley are endless: Put it in soups, substitute it for potatoes or rice, or make it a main ingredient in salads, soups or casseroles.

- ***Brown Rice*** — Rice without the bran removed—is the best choice among the different types of rice. Brown rice, long grain, short grain and converted are some of the more common varieties. Converted rice, also known as parboiled rice, has been steamed under pressure to force nutrients from the bran and germ into the inner grain. The bran and germ are then removed, and the rice is dried and packaged. Enriched rice, on the other hand, has had certain nutrients added to it.

  Brown rice is a better choice than white rice because of its fiber content and nutritional value. White rice has had the bran removed in the refining process.

  Practically anything can be added to rice before or after cooking: chopped vegetables, nuts, dried fruits and an endless array of spices and herbs are just a few.

- ***Buckwheat Groats*** — Buckwheat seeds are called groats, and cooked or roasted groats are called kasha. Kasha is served as a cooked cereal or as a potato substitute.

- ***Bulgur*** — This is a whole wheat berry that is parboiled, dried and broken up. It cooks quickly in only 5 to 10 minutes.

  Because of the pre-cooked and dried condition, the bulgur kernels are quite hard and crystalline in form and may be stored satisfactorily for much longer periods than regular wheat or other cereals. Store in a cool, dry place. Part of the germ is on the wheat and it can become rancid in high temperatures and humidity.

- ***Couscous*** — These are precooked hard-cracked granules of semolina wheat. They can be cooked quickly by a soak-and-steam method, or with a couscousiere, a steamer made specifically for couscous. Sometimes the little grains of couscous tend to stick together, which is why it is steamed instead of boiled. If after cooking they become sticky or gummy, grains can be separated with a fork or your hands.

- ***Cornmeal*** — Ground corn, also called polenta.

- ***Whole Grain Flours*** — Whole wheat, rye, cracked wheat, buckwheat, and stone ground.

Cooking Tips

- Whole grains are more perishable than refined varieties because of the oil in the germ. They are best stored in a cool, dry place to prevent spoilage. They may be refrigerated or kept in your freezer if you plan to store them longer than a month.

- Most whole grain products require more cooking time than the refined grains. As an example, brown rice requires three times the cooking time of white.

- When cooking grains, follow these steps: Rinse the grain in cold water and drain well. Bring water to a boil (stock or milk may be used instead). Pour grain in slowly, stirring as you do, and add salt (1/4 to 1/2 teaspoon per cup of grain). Let the water come to a boil again, then turn the heat down to the lowest possible temperature. Cook slowly until all the water is absorbed.

  If you have cooked the grain the full time and it still seems hard or tough, add a little boiling water, cover and continue cooking. Do not stir it any more than absolutely necessary or it will be gummy. Be sure not to lift the cover while the grain is cooking—steam will escape and the grain might stick.

- When cooking brown rice, remember to first wash the raw rice well and drain. Place it in a saucepan with enough room for the rice to triple in volume. Add twice as much boiling water as rice and return it to a boil. Cover and reduce heat to the lowest point possible. Let the rice cook for 45 minutes. Do not stir because stirring makes rice pasty. Remove from heat. Let it stand several minutes and the rice will steam and dry even more.

  For a slightly different taste, before cooking stir washed rice in a dry saucepan over medium heat until the grain is dry and lightly toasted. This will enhance the nutty flavor. (Don't add salt until after the rice is cooked; it tends to harden the kernels.)

- For a brown rice pilaf, follow the directions for brown rice, but begin by sauteeing a chopped onion, some mushrooms and the washed grain in a tablespoon of broth or oil. Cook, stirring often, until the onion is limp and the grain is dry. Now add boiling water and proceed as usual. If you wish, add boiling meat broth or vegetable broth, tomato juice or a tablespoon of curry powder to the water.

- Wild rice is not really rice, but rather the seed from a grass that grows in water. The only thing it has in common with domestic rice is that they both grow in shallow water. When purchasing wild rice, look for seeds that are fairly consistent in size, with a limited amount of broken pieces in the pack.

  Wild rice will vary in color from brownish and black tint to all shades of dark brown and a very rich dark black color. The flavor should not vary significantly in the different colors, but there will be a difference in cooking times. The darker the rice the longer it will take to cook. Cook until most of the grains curl and pop, but do not overcook wild rice or it will be soft and lose its texture.

  Wild rice is best stored in a cool place, preferably a refrigerator. It has an indefinite shelf life and can be stored 5 to 10 years in a cool, dry place.

- Bulgur and rice are cooked in the same manner. Bulgur can also be eaten uncooked by soaking it in water for several hours. It doubles its dry volume upon cooking or soaking. Do not wash bulgur before, nor rinse after cooking. Use any liquid remaining in the pan after cooking, because it contains valuable minerals and vitamins.

  Do not lift the lid while bulgur is cooking. It does not need to be stirred. Bulgur continues to expand (swell) even after cooking time as long as moisture is available. It may be cooked and stored in a refrigerator for future use.

- To cook couscous: Place couscous in a bowl and pour water over it (1 1/2 cups couscous to 3 cups water). Let sit for 10 to 15 minutes until the water is absorbed. The couscous will now be soft; fluff it with a fork or with your hands. Place the couscous in a colander, sieve, or the top part of a couscousiere above the cooking liquid, making sure the bottom of the colander does not touch the liquid. Seal off the space between the colander and the pot with a towel or cheesecloth. Cover and bring the liquid to a boil. Let steam for 10 minutes, then remove the couscous from the pot and place in a large bowl. Adjust the seasonings and serve at once.

COOKING TIMES AND PROPORTIONS FOR DINNER GRAINS			
Grain (1 cup dry measure)	**Water (cups)**	**Cooking Time (minutes)**	**Yield (cups)**
Barley	3	60-75	3½
Brown Rice	2	45-50	3
Buckwheat (Kasha)	2	15-20	2½
Bulgur Wheat	2	15-20	4 cups
Oats, rolled (old fashioned)	2	10-15	1-2/3
Cracked Wheat	2	20-25	2½
Millet	3	30-45	3½
Coarse Corn Meal (Polenta)	4	25-30	3
Wild Rice	3	60 or more	4

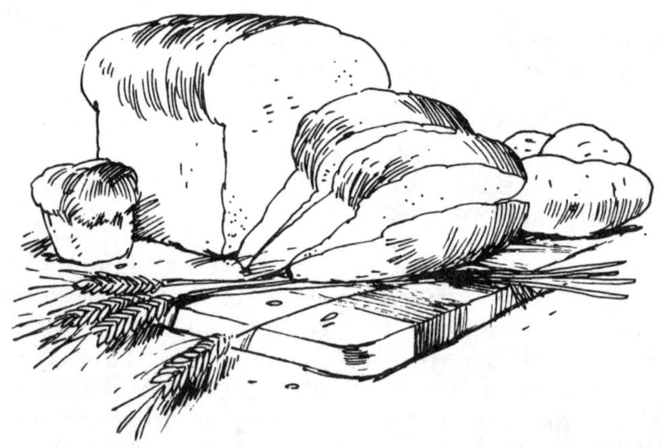

Flours and Breads

Shopping Tips

- Choose breads, cereals and crackers made from grains that retain their natural, fibrous coatings. For whole grain breads, look for whole grain, whole wheat, cracked wheat, stone ground, whole meal or rye flour as the first or second ingredient on the label.
- Buy whole wheat or whole grain flour (or unbleached flour if you use white flour). "Flour" or "wheat flour" on an ingredients list usually refers to bleached white flour.

- Unbleached flour is missing the bran and germ but has escaped the final bleaching process, which destroys even more of the vitamins.

- Of the 22 nutrients removed during milling, enriched flour has only some of them replaced: the B vitamins, vitamin D, calcium, and iron salts. Whole wheat or whole grain flour has had little of the fiber and nutrients removed during milling.

- For a healthier breakfast, eat more bagels, muffins, and pita bread instead of doughnuts and pastries. Making your own muffins or quick bread allows you to reduce the amount of fat even more. Keep your margarine soft to allow for thinner spreading.

Cooking Tips

- Since whole wheat flour is bulkier than white flour, remember the following when using whole wheat flour:

  For every cup of white flour in a recipe:

  USE 1 cup of whole wheat flour minus 2 tablespoons. Decrease the amount of oil called for in the recipe by 1 tablespoon and increase the liquid called for by 1 to 2 tablespoons. (This is not necessary if a finely ground whole wheat flour is used.)

  OR USE 1/2 cup white and 1/2 cup whole wheat flour.

  OR USE 3/4 cup white and 1/4 cup wheatgerm or 1/4 cup 100 percent bran.

- Since whole wheat flour spoils rapidly, store it in a freezer or refrigerator.

- In the baking of bread, yeast needs a small amount of carbohydrate (sugar or starch) as food. Salt controls the rising action of yeast. If salt is omitted, the rising rate may change. Temperatures above 115 F destroy yeast, so liquid added to a yeast mixture should be cooler than that.

  Dough must be mixed or kneaded thoroughly to develop the gluten that gives it structure and distributes liquid evenly. It should also be covered with a towel and left to rise in a warm place (80-85 F) free of drafts. To test if the dough has risen enough, press two fingers into the surface. If the indentation remains, the dough is ready to be baked.

  When kneading dough, keep it from sticking by greasing your fingertips and lightly flouring the board. Use a little more flour as needed, but be careful not to add too much. Excess flour makes a drier, heavier bread.

A tin with a dull finish is best for baking. Remove baked products from baking pans immediately after taking them out of the oven.

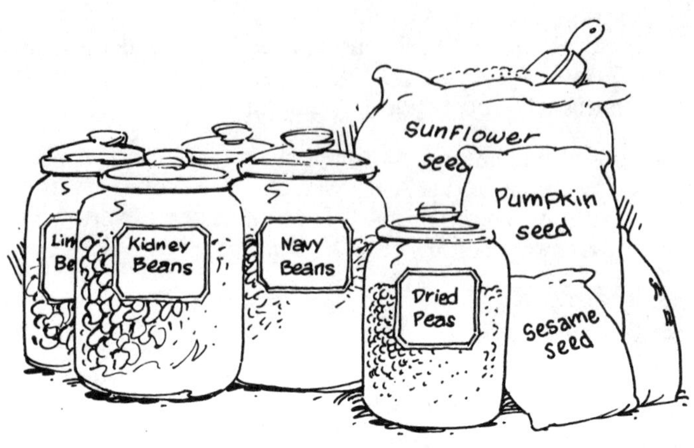

Legumes

"Legume" is a general term referring to dried beans, peas and lentils. These foods rank high on the list of sources of iron, zinc, magnesium, phosphorus, thiamine, B6, niacin and folacin, and they are fair sources of calcium and riboflavin.

Legumes are often classified as a meat substitute because of their high protein content. An average serving, about 3/4 cup cooked, supplies approximately 11 grams of protein, which is 18 percent of the daily RDA for protein. Fiber is also found in cooked or canned dried beans (lima, kidney, navy, pinto), dried peas and lentils, all varieties of nuts, and pumpkin, sesame and sunflower seeds.

One reason legumes are not used more frequently is the difficulty in digesting them—undigestible carbohydrate in beans leads to intestinal flatulence (gas). To prevent gas problems, increase the amount of legumes in your diet gradually. Your intestine will adapt to the new carbohydrate source over time, thus decreasing gas production. Also try different types of legumes because everybody has a different tolerance to each variety.

In addition, remember to cook legumes well. Cooking for a long time at a lower heat may help to reduce their flatulence-causing properties. If you use the soaking method of cooking beans, discarding the water before cooking may reduce digestive symptoms. But be aware that you will also be discarding some of the vitamins and minerals.

Start with lentils, split peas and lima beans—these are the most easily digested legumes. And begin with small servings to give your body a chance to adjust.

Legumes are another category of food mistakenly thought of as fattening. Because of their high fiber content, they tend to be very filling—an added bonus for those on a low calorie diet.

Beans, peas and lentils are a primary source of protein in much of the world. By themselves, however, they are an incomplete protein, meaning that they lack or are low in certain amino acids needed by the body to form protein. Nine amino acids cannot be made by the body and must come from food. Beans, with the exception of soybeans, are deficient in two of these amino acids, tryptophan and methionine. Their strengths are the amino acids lysine and isoleucine. However, whole grains, wheat, nuts, seeds and dairy products are rich in tryptophan and methionine, and weak in lysine and isoleucine, so when combined with legumes they offer the value of a complete protein. Soybean protein is a complete protein; in fact, its amino acid pattern is close to that of milk.

The three main sources of vegetable proteins are legumes, grains, nuts and seeds. Small amounts of meat, poultry, fish, egg whites and dairy products can be added to plant proteins to make them complete.

In the diagram on the next page, arrows indicate foods that may be eaten together to complement (or complete) the proteins. This diagram will help you plan meals around complementary proteins in two ways: either combine two or more foods from the vegetable proteins (boxes on the outside) or combine a vegetable source with a low-fat animal-protein source (box in the center).

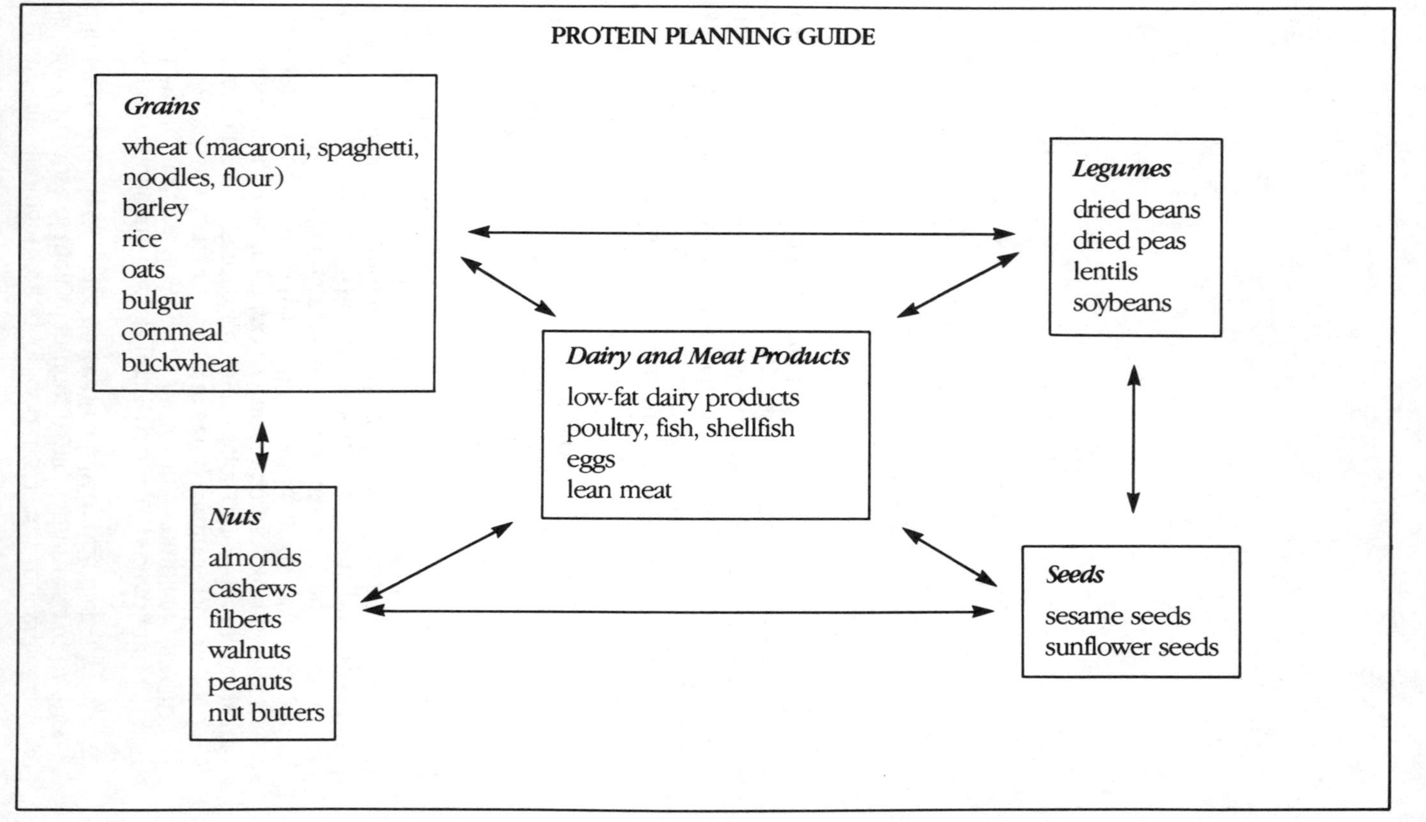
PROTEIN PLANNING GUIDE
Grains
wheat (macaroni, spaghetti, noodles, flour)
barley
rice
oats
bulgur
cornmeal
buckwheat
Legumes
dried beans
dried peas
lentils
soybeans
Dairy and Meat Products
low-fat dairy products
poultry, fish, shellfish
eggs
lean meat
Nuts
almonds
cashews
filberts
walnuts
peanuts
nut butters
Seeds
sesame seeds
sunflower seeds

Meals with vegetable protein in place of meat, poultry or fish can be low in fat unless they contain a lot of high-fat dairy products. In addition, they are sources of variety in the diet, besides being economical and highly nutritive when adequate in protein. The following table gives you some comparison of various protein sources.

PROTEIN SOURCE COMPARISON

Food	Amount	Protein (gms)	Fat (gms)	Calories
Meat	3 oz. cooked, lean boneless sirloin	24	10	195
Cheese	3 oz. cheddar cheese	21	27	336
Legumes	1½ cups cooked navy beans	23	2	314

Most people do not want to eliminate animal products completely, but you can see it isn't necessary to eat animal protein at every meal or even every day to have sufficient protein in your diet.

Shopping Tips

- When purchasing legumes, look for beans, peas and lentils with a bright color, uniform size, and no visible damage. Legumes should be stored in tightly covered containers in a dry, cool place (50 to 70 F). They will keep their quality for several months. Do not mix older legumes with newly purchased ones; this will result in uneven cooking, since older legumes take longer to cook than fresher ones.

  The following is a list of legumes and their uses:

  Black beans can be used in thick soups and oriental and Mediterranean dishes.

  Black-eyed peas (or cow peas) are small, oval-shaped beans that are creamy white with a small black spot on one side. They are popular in Southern and soul food cookery. Serve them as a main dish vegetable.

  Garbanzo beans (chick peas) have a nut-like flavor, which makes them useful in dips and main dishes. Commonly pickled in vinegar and oil for salads and in Middle Eastern dishes, they are often served cold for snacking.

Great Northern beans, similar to pea beans but larger, are used in soups, main dishes and home-baked bean dishes.

Kidney beans are red and shaped like a kidney and are frequently used in Mexican dishes, especially chili.

Lentils are light brown and disk-shaped, about the size of a pea. They cook in only 30 to 45 minutes and do not need soaking. Lentils team up well with other vegetables, grains, meat, or in soups, gravies or stews. Serve them chilled as a salad on a lettuce bed.

Lima beans are broad and flat and come in small and large sizes. They are excellent as a vegetable casserole ingredient and in soup.

Navy beans is a general name for all small white beans, Great Northern and pea beans.

Pea beans are small, oval and white, a favorite for homemade baked beans, soups and casseroles.

Pinto beans are a relative of the kidney bean. They are beige colored with speckles. Use them as you would kidney beans.

Red beans and pink beans are members of the kidney bean family with a more delicate flavor. Both are used in chili and Mexican dishes.

Soybeans can be used just as any other bean. They are light tan and round, like a large pea. Used in stews, casseroles and soups, soybeans are made into many products—tofu, soymilk and meat substitutes.

Dry split peas, available in green and yellow, have the skin removed by mechanical processing. They are best known for their use in split pea soup but combine well with other foods. You can cook them in a relatively short period of time. They do not require soaking, so they can be cooked along with rice or other grains for a protein-rich dish.

Dry whole peas can be served plain, boiled and seasoned, with meats, or in dips, soups, casseroles, croquettes, and even souffles. They must be soaked before cooking.

Cooking Tips

- Beans come direct from the fields, so you should rinse them well in cold water and sort through them, removing any visible stones or other debris. Most beans and peas, except for lentils and split peas, should be soaked in cold water for at least eight hours or overnight before cooking.

- Soybeans should be refrigerated during presoaking to prevent fermentation. Lentils and split peas need only to be cleaned before cooking.
- Instead of overnight soaking, you can save some time by bringing the beans and water to a boil and covering them tightly. Simmer for two minutes, remove from the heat and allow to stand for two hours.
- Cover beans with water, bring them to a boil and let them simmer until tender. Check occasionally and add more water if needed. Don't add salt, oil or spices until the beans are tender, or they won't cook. Keep the pot partially covered at all times; they usually boil over if covered tightly.
- Don't mix different kinds of beans when cooking unless you are using a crock pot.
- The amount of water recommended can vary, but keep beans covered with liquid at all times.
- Allow for expansion of legumes when cooking. Depending on the kind, 1 cup of dried legumes yields 2 to 2 3/4 cups cooked.
- Cooking time is also variable. If you are cooking beans for a salad or any dish in which they should remain intact, cook them just until tender. For soups, they can be cooked a good deal longer.
- Canned beans and peas are convenient if time is a concern. Rinse them well to remove added salt.

COOKING TIMES AND PROPORTIONS FOR BEANS			
Beans (1 cup dry measure)	Water (cups)	Cooking Time (hours)	Yield (cups)
Black beans	4	1½-2	2
Black-eyed peas	3	1-2	2
Garbanzos	4	3-4	2
Great Northern beans	3½	2	2
Kidney beans	3	1½	2
Lentils & split peas	3	1	2¼
Lima	2	1½	1¼
Baby lima	2	1½	1¾
Pinto beans	3	2-2½	2
Small red beans	3	3	2
Small white beans (navy, etc.)	3	1½	2
Soybeans	4	2-3 or more	2
Soy grits	2	15-20 minutes	2

■ Pressure cooking can be an advantage with legumes because of shortness in cooking times. It also yields a more tender bean. Place the beans in water equal to three to four times their volume and bring to a boil in the pressure cooker. Cover and bring them to 15 pounds pressure, cooking them according to the timetable below. Cool the pressure cooker immediately under cold running water. Open the cooker and drain the stock from the beans.

Soaking or precooking saves a little time, but with pressure cooking it really isn't necessary. Lentils and peas (split or black-eyed) tend to foam when cooking, so if you are using a pressure cooker, do so with caution. Sometimes adding a little oil to the mixture keeps the foam down.

TIMETABLE FOR PRESSURE COOKING UNSOAKED BEANS	
	Cooking Time (minutes)
Black beans, kidney, black-eyed peas, pinto, soybeans	20-25
Mung beans, small red beans	30-35
Garbanzo	40-45
Lentils, split peas	10-15

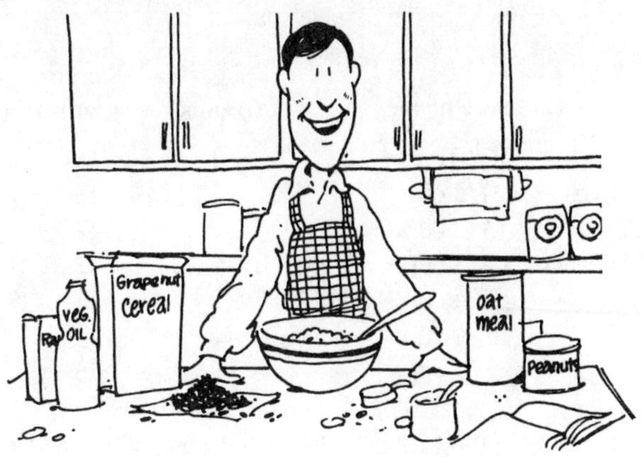

Cereals

Cereals make excellent breakfast choices. They are in most cases complex carbohydrates and valuable sources of fiber in the diet.

Be aware, however, that some cereals contain a significant amount of sugar. A U.S. Department of Agriculture Human Nutrition Center study showed only three of 62 ready-to-serve breakfast cereals contained less than 1 percent sugar. Two contained more than 50 percent sugar.

Here is a list of cereals with their percentages of sugar and grams of sugar as reported in the *Journal of Food Science*, 1980.

SUGAR, STARCH AND FIBER CONTENT OF CEREALS
(Based on a 70 calorie, 15 gram carbohydrate service size)

Cereal	Serving Size	Sugar* (grams)	Starch (grams)	Dietary Fiber** (grams)
Cereals containing approximately 10 percent or less sugar:*				
Oats, Oatmeal	1/2 cup cooked	—	12	2.9
Puffed Wheat	3/4 cup	—	13	3.4
Shredded Wheat	1 biscuit	—	14	2.8
Ralstons	1/2 cup cooked	1	14	2.1
Cheerios	1 cup	1	13	2.5
Chex, Corn	2/3 cup	1	15	2.6
Chex, Wheat	1/2 cup	1	13	2
Corn Flakes	2/3 cup	1	15	2.6

continued

Cereal	Serving Size	Sugar* (grams)	Starch (grams)	Dietary Fiber** (grams)
Grape Nuts	3 Tbsp.	1	13	2.7
Nutri-Grains	1/2 cup	1	13	2
Corn Bran	1/2 cup	2	12	4.4
Grape Nut Flakes	2/3 cup	2	12	2.5
Oat Bran	1/4 cup	2	7	5.3
Total	3/4 cup	2	13	2.5
Wheaties	3/4 cup	2	13	2.6
Cereals containing approximately 10 to 30 percent sugar:				
Bran Chex	1/2 cup	4	10	4.1
40% Bran Flakes	2/3 cup	4	11	3
Most	1/3 cup	4	8	3
All Bran	1/3 cup	5	7	9
Cracklin' Bran	1/3 cup	5	5	3
Frosted Mini-Whts.	2½ biscuits	5	10	1.3
Honey Bran	2/3 cup	5	10	2.4
Raisin Bran	2/3 cup	8 (4 from sugar 4 from raisins)	12	3.4
Cereals containing 30 to 40 percent sugar:				
Wheat and Raisin Chex	1/2 cup	6 (3 from sugar 3 from raisins)	10	2
Bran Buds	1/3 cup	8	6	8
Cereals containing 40 percent or more sugar:				
Frosted Rice, Sugar Frosted Flakes, Cocoa Puffs, Lucky Charms, Quisp	1/2 cup	7	9	—

continued

Cereal	Serving Size	Sugar* (grams)	Starch (grams)	Dietary Fiber** (grams)
Sugar Corn Pops, Trix Chocolate or Strawberry Crazy Cow, Cocoa Krispies, Franken Berry, Count Chocula, Boo Berry, Cookie Crisp, Cap'n Crunch	2/3 cup	8	8	—
Cereals containing 54-55 percent sugar:				
Apple Jacks, Fruit Loops	2/3 cup	9	8	—
Sugar Smacks	1/2 cup	10	6	—

*Source: USDA Nutrient Composition Laboratory. Nutrition Institute, Human Nutrition Center, Bettsville, MD. Journal of Food Science 45 (1): 138-141, 1980.

**Source: Anderson JW, Chen WL, Sieling B: Plant Fiber in Foods. HCF Diabetes Research Foundation, Inc., Lexington, Kentucky; Kellogg's; Ralston Purina.

Shopping Tips

- Granola is a heavy, chewy dry cereal made with whole grains, nuts, seeds, raisins, honey and oil. Commercial granola's nutritious ingredients, however, are usually canceled out by other not so healthy ingredients. Most of the granola cereals are prepared with palm or coconut oil, which are even more saturated than lard. These two oils are used to prolong the freshness of the product. Others contain partially hydrogenated peanut, soy or cottonseed oils, which are moderately saturated. Only Vita Crunch uses unhydrogenated soy oil.

  Commercial granolas contain about 8 grams (2 teaspoons) of sugar per ounce. Brown sugar and honey add empty calories. The total sugar content of granola cereals ranges from 22 to 32 percent of their dry weight.

A one-ounce serving of granola (1/4 cup) contains 140 calories and barely covers the bottom of your bowl. A more realistic serving is 1/2 or 3/4 cup. If you eat a 1-ounce serving of shredded wheat, you get 3/4 cup of cereal at 1/4 of granola's calories for the same volume of cereal. One ounce of Cheerios is 1 1/4 cups and has 1/6 the calories of 1 1/4 cups of granola with very little fat and almost no sugar. Using granola cereals for snacking is not a good idea if you are trying to watch your calorie intake.

Granola cereals are usually not high in vitamins and minerals, because they are not fortified or enriched as are other cereal products. Granola contains only about four to eight percent of the U.S. RDA for thiamin, iron, magnesium, copper and zinc. Enriched cereals would be a better source of vitamins and minerals. Most granolas have less dietary fiber than most people think—only 1.8 to 4.8 percent.

SUGAR AND CALORIC CONTENT OF GRANOLA CEREALS

Cereal (1/4 cup)	Total Sugar (grams)	Table Sugar (grams)	Total Calories
General Mills Nature Valley Granola-fruit and nuts	28.4	19.4	All are approximately 140 calories
General Foods C.W. Post-plain	24.1	19.1	
General Foods C.W. Post-raisin	27.2	19.0	
Pet Heartland-coconut	21.6	18.1	
Quaker Oats 100% Natural-apple and cinnamon	23.44	17.9	
Quaker Oats 100% Natural-brown sugar and honey	21.4	17.5	
Kellogg Country Morning	29.7	17.3	
General Mills Nature Valley Granola cinnamon and raisin	23.2	17.2	
Familia	22.6	15.4	
Quaker Oats 100% Natural-raisins and dates	26.1	14.7	

- What about granola bars? Choose a granola bar with the least amount of sugar. Some granola bars have 40 percent of their calories as complex carbohydrates, 20 percent as sugar and 35 percent as fat (Quaker and General Mills). Others may have only 25 percent of their calories as complex carbohydrates and 50 percent as sugar. (Candy bars are about 40 percent sugar and 53 percent fat.) One granola bar will usually have about 130 calories, 15 to 20 grams of carbohydrate (3-10 grams sugar), 2 grams of protein, and 5 grams of fat.

  Now, however, chocolate chips have been added to some granola bars and the bars coated with chocolate. As a result, sugar or products containing sugar have become the main ingredient. They now contain fat from hydrogenated vegetable oil as well as chocolate, both primarily saturated fats. Although these granola bars look like candy bars, have approximately the same number of calories as candy bars, and taste like exceptionally sweet candy bars, they are not sold with the candy bars; instead they are in the cereal section!

- Some cereals can also contribute sodium to the diet. Those which may be of concern to individuals who need to restrict sodium because of health problems are listed below:

CEREALS THAT ARE CONCENTRATED SOURCES OF SODIUM

	Sodium (milligrams) Per One-Cup Serving
Kellogg All-Bran	930
General Foods Grape Nuts	840
Kellogg Cracklin' Bran	660
General Foods 40% Bran Flakes	450
General Mills Golden Grahams	430
Kellogg Raisin Bran	370

Low sodium choices are: **Puffed Rice**
Puffed Wheat
Shredded Wheat
Cooked cereals, prepared without salt (except the mix-and-eat variety)

Cooking Tips

- The traditional breakfast of bacon, eggs, and toast with butter is high in fat, calories and sodium. Fruit or fruit juice, toast, English muffins or bagels with small amounts of margarine, and cereal with skim milk are healthy alternatives.
- Make a hot cereal or choose a ready-to-serve cold cereal that is not sugar-coated. When selecting ready-to-cook hot cereals, remember that instant cereals are more refined and are usually lower in fiber.
- If you're disappointed that commercial granolas are not the best way to fill a healthy breakfast bowl or use for a snack, make it yourself! That way you can choose the best ingredients for your needs and cut back on others. Homemade granola can contain a less saturated vegetable oil, such as corn, safflower or soy. You can also cut down on the amount of oil to minimize the fat and reduce or eliminate sugar and honey.

  Making granola is easy. Coat raw cereal grain (usually rolled oats) with a very small amount of oil and toast them until dry. Make sure you use only a small amount of oil—just enough to make the oats crunchy and tasty. If you skip the oil, the cereal will be too hard to chew. Don't add raisins before baking or they will also be hard.
- If granola is a big hit in your house, try making the following recipe. It is used at Camp Needlepoint, a camp for children with diabetes.

HOMEMADE GRANOLA

Ingredients (for 15 1/2 servings)

4 cups oatmeal (quick type)
1 cup chopped peanuts (no skins)
1/2 cup Grape Nuts
1/2 cup bran (unprocessed, uncooked)
1/3 cup vegetable oil
Sugar substitute to equal 1/2 cup sugar (Dry sugar substitute works best.)
1/2 cup wheat germ
1/2 cup raisins

Directions:

1. Spread the oatmeal on a cookie sheet and heat in oven at 350 F for 10 minutes.
2. Combine all but the last three ingredients. Bake on an ungreased cookie

sheet or pan for 20 minutes, stirring once to brown oatmeal evenly.

3. Add wheat germ, raisins and sugar substitute.
4. Refrigerate in glass jars or plastic containers.

One serving (1/2 cup) contains 140 calories, 15 grams carbohydrate, 5 grams protein, 7 grams fat, and 46 milligrams sodium. (If you are on an exchange meal plan, one serving equals 1 Bread Exchange and 1 Fat Exchange.)

For a homemade granola bar try the following recipe:

"YOUR OWN" GRANOLA BARS

Ingredients (for 30 bars)

3 1/2 cups toasted quick oats
1 cup raisins (optional)
1/2 cup chopped nuts (optional)
2/3 cup margarine, melted
1/4 cup brown sugar (firmly packed)
1/2 cup honey
1 egg (beaten)
1/2 teaspoon vanilla
1/2 teaspoon salt

Directions:

1. Spread quick oats on a cookie sheet and bake in a 350 F oven for 15 to 20 minutes, or until light golden brown.
2. Combine all ingredients and mix well. Place firmly into a well-greased 12 1/2 inch by 10 1/2 inch pan.
3. Bake in 350 F oven for 20 minutes.
4. Cool. Cut into bars. Store in tightly covered container in cool dry place or in refrigerator.

One serving contains 115 calories, 15 grams of carbohydrate, 12 grams of protein, 6 grams of fat, and 90 milligrams of sodium (1 bread and 1 fat exchange).

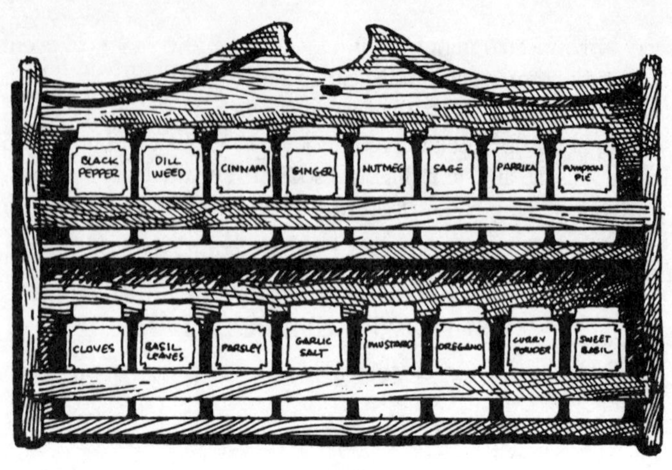

5

SHAKE THE SALT HABIT: BAN THE SHAKER!

Another key to opening the door to healthy nutrition is to avoid excessive salt (sodium). Table salt is 40 percent sodium and 60 percent chloride. There is increasing evidence that current levels of sodium intake may be one of the contributing causes of high blood pressure in people who are genetically susceptible. About 20 percent of the population is thought to be susceptible, but the risk for older people is 40 percent. (Blood pressure is the force exerted on the walls of the arteries as blood flows through them. High blood pressure is known as hypertension.)

For many people, weight loss or a reduction in sodium intake will lower blood pressure. Individuals who take medication to control blood pressure should be particularly careful of the amount of sodium included in their diet. Anyone with high blood pressure should be under close medical supervision.

Desire for salt does not come from a basic need but rather through an acquired taste. One of the best ways to cut back on salt is to simply take the shaker off the table. At first foods may seem less tasty, and it may take from three to six weeks to adjust. But you will be amazed to discover that some bland foods will acquire unexpected flavor resources, and a new world of sharpened senses will open up. You will also become aware of the way salt dominates the flavor of many processed foods.

The average intake of salt ranges from about 6 to 18 grams a day. However, the human requirement for sodium is only about 1/4 gram per day, which is 1/10 of a teaspoon. A goal for sodium is to reduce your salt intake to about 5 grams or 1 teaspoon of salt per day. One teaspoon of salt contains 2,300 milligrams of sodium.

The salt shaker is not the only source of sodium. Many foods from fast-food restaurants and many "convenience" processed foods are laced with salt and other sodium-containing compounds: sodium benzoate, monosodium glutamate, sodium nitrate, etc.

To decide whether to cut back on the amount of salt in recipes, you need to calculate how much of the total amount of salt will be in each serving. Although one teaspoon of salt contains 2,300 milligrams of sodium, omitting the salt from an eight-person casserole that calls for one teaspoon of salt may not be worth the taste change, because each serving will contain less than 300 milligrams of sodium. This may also be true for the baking soda and salt used in home baking; the amount of sodium per serving isn't likely to be a problem unless you are on a very restrictive diet.

The comparison below gives you some idea of what happens to the sodium content in the processing of food!

SODIUM CONTENT:
NATURAL VS. PROCESSED FOODS

	Amount	Sodium Content (milligrams)
Milk	1 cup	122
Processed cheese	1 oz.	425
Vegetables, fresh or frozen	1 cup	2
Vegetables, canned	1 cup	385
Pork chop	3 oz.	59
Ham or bologna	3 oz.	1,114
Hamburger, lean	3 oz.	57
Hamburger, fast food	3 oz.	990

Shopping Tips

- Be aware of other sources of sodium in the diet:

  One level teaspoon of salt has 2,300 milligrams of sodium.
  One level teaspoon of baking soda has 1,000 milligrams of sodium.
  One level teaspoon of monosodium glutamate has 750 milligrams of sodium.
  One level teaspoon of baking powder has 329 milligrams of sodium.

  The following are the most common sodium compounds added to foods: "soda" and "sodium" (symbol "Na"). But don't worry about sodium saccharin, di-sodium phosphate, sodium alginate, propionate, benzoate, sulfite or hydroxide, because they contain little sodium.

- The FDA is strongly encouraging food makers to do four things: 1) label for sodium content, 2) change cooking directions so adding salt is optional, 3) reduce the amount of sodium in processed foods, and 4) offer many more low-sodium or salt-free products.

- Federal law requires that by July 1986 food processors must specify the sodium content of products that carry nutritional labeling. Information has been provided for calories, protein, carbohydrate, fat, and some minerals and vitamins. The sodium content will be given in milligrams of sodium. Foods without nutritional labeling are exempt from the sodium requirement. It is estimated that more than half the packaged processed food sales regulated by the FDA will have sodium content information on their labels.

  The FDA has established guidelines for sodium label claims as well:

  Sodium free: to describe foods that contain less than 5 milligrams of sodium per serving.
  Very low sodium: 35 milligrams or less of sodium per serving.
  Low sodium: 140 milligrams or less of sodium per serving.
  Reduced sodium: foods that have had their sodium content reduced by 75 percent. In this instance, the food label will need to provide data comparing the sodium content of the product with that of the food it is replacing.
  Unsalted, no salt added, without added salt: these terms can only be used if no salt has been added to a product that is normally processed with salt.

  In addition, foods making any of the above claims will have to list milligrams of sodium per serving on the label. The FDA developed these terms to promote consistency in sodium labeling and to reduce consumer confusion.

- Reduce purchasing of foods with visible salt such as pretzels, potato chips, corn chips and salted nuts. Also limit pickled foods, ham, bacon, smoked meats, pickles, pickle relish, seasoned salts, olives, sauerkraut, processed cheese, "fast foods," "convenience" foods (ready-prepared foods—canned, frozen, packaged entrees, sauces, etc.).

Here are some examples of sodium content in high salt foods:

SODIUM CONTENT OF HIGH SALT FOODS

Food Product	Sodium (milligrams)
One-half package chicken-coating mix	1,300
"Fast Food" hamburger and french fries	1,300
One tablespoon soy sauce	1,300
One-half 10-inch pizza	1,250
One frozen TV dinner	1,200
One-cup package macaroni and cheese	1,200
Five ounces luncheon meat or ham	1,050
One frankfurter	1,000
One-half dill pickle	1,000
One bouillon cube	1,000
One cup canned or packaged soup	900
Three-fourths cup canned tuna, sardines, etc.	850
Two-thirds cup baked beans	750
Four large olives or one-half cup sauerkraut	500
One cup instant mashed potatoes	485
Eight cracker squares	480
One ounce processed cheddar cheese	420
One cup canned vegetables	385

- Choose snacks such as vegetable sticks, unsalted nuts and popcorn (unsalted). Cut back on salty snacks, such as potato and corn chips, and salty crackers and nuts, which are high in saturated fats and calories too. They can make you thirsty for those high-calorie soft drinks. See suggestions for healthy snacks on pages 161-162.

- Regular sodas and diet sodas sweetened with sodium saccharin vary in the amount of sodium contained, an average being approximately 35 to 60 milligrams per 12-ounce can. One or two cans a day will not be a significant source of sodium.

- Read labels for sodium compounds and sodium content in processed foods. Replace such foods with homemade varieties whenever possible. Commercial mayonnaise and salad dressings, for example, may contain high levels of sodium.

Cooking Tips

To shake the salt habit:

- Use a light hand on your salt shaker. Cut down on the salt you add during cooking and at meals.

- Experiment with herbs and spices as alternatives to high sodium condiments, such as soy sauce, steak sauce, catsup and seasoned salts. Substitute tasty vegetables such as onion or green pepper. Use lemon juice or spices such as thyme, oregano, garlic, curry, cinnamon, chili or tarragon. Garlic salt, onion salt and celery salt all add additional salt to your daily intake, so select pure herbs and spices—minus the salt. Onion powder or garlic powder may be used. And reach for the pepper! Or try the new salt-free lemon-herb mixtures available in supermarkets.

- Use flavors that add special zest to foods: fresh herbs such as parsley, tarragon, finely chopped garlic and fresh grated horseradish, spices such as curry and chili powders, powdered mustard (made into a paste with water), hot pepper flakes or a generous grinding of black pepper.

- These recipes can be placed in shakers and used instead of salt:

  Saltless Surprise
  2 tsp. garlic powder
  1 tsp. basil
  1 tsp. anise seed
  1 tsp. oregano
  1 tsp. powdered lemon rind or dry lemon juice

  Put ingredients into blender and mix well. Store in glass container, label well and add rice to prevent caking.

Pungent Salt Substitute

3 tsp. basil
2 tsp. savory (summer savory is best)
2 tsp. celery seed
2 tsp. ground cumin seed
2 tsp. sage
1 tsp. lemon thyme
2 tsp. marjoram

Mix well and then powder with mortar and pestle.

- Season stews, gravies and soups with herbs, vinegar or lemon juice instead of salt, or add one teaspoon of prepared mustard per cup of liquid, or a few hearty dashes of Angostura bitters.

- Cut back on use of luncheon meats, ham, bacon, frankfurters, sausage, and other smoked, pickled or salted foods. Instead, use fresh meats, poultry and fish.

- Use fresh or frozen fish instead of canned or dried varieties.

- Avoid or use these seasonings sparingly, because most of them contain one or more sodium compounds:

Celery salt	Meat/vegetable extracts	Worcestershire sauce
Garlic salt	Barbecue sauces	Olives, pickles, relishes
Onion salt	Meat sauces	Cooking wine
Catsup	Meat tenderizers	Prepared mustard
Chili sauce	Commercial bouillon	Sea salt
Steak sauce	Soy sauce	

- Salt may be needed in a recipe to cause or control chemical reaction, especially recipes using yeast. You may be able to omit or reduce the amount of salt in baking, but the resulting product may be different from the original. Do some experimenting to see what works.

- Salt substitutes are usually composed of potassium chloride instead of sodium chloride. The potassium often leaves a bitter aftertaste, so it may be better to adjust to the taste of less salt. Light salt is a mixture of potassium chloride and sodium chloride and it does not taste as bitter. Some salt substitutes may affect prescribed drug therapy. Check with your doctor before using them, especially if you are on a restricted diet or are taking any drugs.

- Rinsing commercial foods with plain tap water can cut back significantly on sodium. A one-minute rinse of 6 1/2 ounces of commercially canned tuna will wash away about 75 percent of the sodium. Forty percent of the sodium can be drained from canned vegetables by rinsing for one minute and heating them in tap water instead of the canning liquid.

- Water in which salty products are cooked can be poured off and replaced with fresh water.
- Do not automatically add salt to boiling water when cooking pasta, vegetables and cereals.
- Use flavors that add special zest to foods: fresh herbs such as parsley, tarragon, finely chopped garlic and fresh grated horseradish; and spices such as curry and chili powders, powdered mustard (made into a paste with water), hot pepper flakes or a generous grinding of black pepper.
- Chives, parsley, tarragon, dill and basil accompany most vegetables well. Lemon juice can also be used. Be sure to add lemon juice after cooking or it will toughen vegetables. Cinnamon, ginger, allspice and nutmeg enhance the taste of carrots and winter squash. They provide excellent alternatives to the typical butter and salt routine.
- To flavor meats, poultry and fish, try onion or garlic powder, paprika, parsley, thyme, sage, rosemary, dry mustard or oregano. When using garlic or onion powder, use less than with the salts, because the salt isn't there to take up volume.
- When trying new flavorings, begin by using no more than one or two herbs or spices at a time. Start with small amounts—add 1/4 teaspoon of diced herbs or one teaspoon of chopped seasonings to soups and stews before the last hour of cooking or the flavor will be destroyed. However, mix herbs and spices into cold dressings, dips or marinades at least several hours before serving to "blend" the flavors.

HERB AND SPICE GUIDE FOR FOOD FLAVORING*

Herbs: the leaves, seeds or flowers of aromatic plants. Fresh herbs are preferable. Dried herbs should not be used in cold dishes. Use half as much of a dried herb as you would use of a fresh one.

Spices: the roots, bark, stems, buds, seeds and fruit of aromatic tropical plants.

Herbs and Spices:	**Use in these foods:**
Allspice	Stews, soups, ground meats, barbecue sauce, tomatoes
Almond Extract	Fruits, puddings
Basil	Beef, lamb, seafoods, soups, stews, stewed or fresh tomatoes
Bay Leaves	Meats, poultry, soups, stews, spaghetti dishes
Caraway seeds	Meats, salads, breads, stews, asparagus, cabbage
Chives	Salads, sauces, soups, stews, fish, meats, vegetables
Celery Seed	Meat loaf, cole slaw, soups
Cinnamon	Fruits (especially apples), breads, pork, fish, squash, sweet potatoes
Chili Powder	Ground meats, casseroles, seafood, corn, French dressing
Cloves	Fruits, roasted meats, baked fish, squash
Curry Powder	Lamb, chicken, fish, beef, vegetables
Dill Weed	Soups, salads, fish, meat, chicken, carrots, peas, zucchini
Garlic (not the salt)	Casseroles, meats, salads, vegetables, tomato dishes
Ginger	Chicken, oriental vegetables, fruits
Lemon or Lime Juice	Vegetables, meats, fish, seafoods, salads, fruit
Mace	Hot breads, fruit salads, fish, veal
Marjoram	Lamb, salmon, eggplant, green salads
Mint	Fruit cups, veal, lamb, fish, sauces, green peas
Mustard (dry)	Ground meats, fish, salads, sauces, beans
Nutmeg	Cottage cheese, eggs, fruits, vegetables
Onion (not the salt)	Meats, fish, vegetables, salads, tomatoes
Oregano	Soups, stews, Italian casseroles, steaks, seafoods, tomatoes
Paprika	Chicken, fish, meats, baked potatoes, cole slaw, wax beans
Pepper or Peppercorns	Soups, stews, meats, chicken, vegetables, dressings
Peppermint Extract	Fruits, puddings
Pimento	Salads, vegetable combinations, casseroles
Rosemary	Meats, fish, poultry, dressings, potatoes, peas

Sage	Poultry, meat, stuffings, rice, stews, green beans, tomatoes
Savory	Scrambled eggs, soups, pork, ground meats, vegetables
Sherry (not cooking)	Cream Sherry: Fruits Dry Sherry: Soups, stews
Tarragon	Soups, salads, meats, chicken, greens
Thyme	Chicken, veal, pork, soups, salads, onions, tomatoes
Tumeric	Meats, fish, sauces, rice

Additional flavoring aids: Anise seed, cardamom, cumin, fennel, parsley and parsley flakes, poultry seasoning, vinegar (especially wine and salad vinegars), vermouth, wines.

Microwave tips for spices:

- Sprinkle paprika and parsley flakes on meats for color and "browning effect."
- Sprinkle nutmeg or paprika on breads, custards, or quiches for color.
- Dry fresh herbs (parsley, chives, etc.) between paper toweling for lasting dried herbs.

*Provided by: Nutrition Section — Health Education Department
Park Nicollet Medical Foundation

6

THE CAFFEINE KICK

A nutrition key that may or may not be important for you is to watch caffeine consumption. Caffeine, a widely consumed chemical present in many foods and medicines, is most common in coffee, tea, chocolate, cocoa, soft drinks, and medicines such as cold remedies and pain relievers. Caffeine is a natural substance in plants that are sources of coffee, tea, and the kola nut used in soft drinks and cocoa. (Chocolate and cocoa contain caffeine from cocoa beans.) Caffeine has no taste and can be removed from a product by a chemical process called decaffeination.

Caffeine stimulates the central nervous system, though some individuals are more susceptible to its effects than others. Caffeine in beverages is readily absorbed from the gastrointestinal tract and distributed in the various tissues of the body, passing rapidly into the central nervous system. A "drug dose" of caffeine is considered to be 250 milligrams of caffeine per day (about two to three cups of coffee).

The American Council of Science and Health and the Institute of Food Technologists have concluded that on the basis of current scientific evidence, caffeine consumed in foods, beverages, and over-the-counter drugs is not a threat to the health of most Americans. However, some people who consume large amounts may experience chronic headaches, sleep disturbances, rapid heartbeat, anxiety, stomach upset, restlessness and nervousness, all resulting from the stimulation of the central nervous system. These adverse effects may occur at daily consumption levels at or above 4 to 5 cups of brewed coffee, 10 to 12 cups of instant coffee, 10 to 12 cups of tea, 15 12-ounce servings of caffeinated soft drinks, or six doses of certain over-the-counter drug preparations.

Caffeine is of special concern in children because of their body size and weight. For an adult, one cup of coffee or cola would provide about 1 gram of caffeine per kilogram of body weight. In a young child, a cup of chocolate or candy bar would give the same proportion of caffeine to body weight. In fact, a child drinking a can of cola, Dr. Pepper or Mountain Dew has a caffeine intake per kilogram of body weight comparable to an adult drinking 4 cups of coffee. Restlessness, irritability, sleeplessness and nervousness are reported in children and teenagers consuming large amounts of cola beverages and chocolate.

A syndrome called "caffeinism" or "coffee nerves," which has been likened to an anxiety neurosis, has been reported to disappear in some people who eliminate caffeine-containing foods and beverages. "Excessive" caffeine intake is defined as more than 1,000 milligrams per day, or 10 cups of strong brewed coffee. Because caffeine's effects are highly individual, it may cause problems for some people but not others. People who are used to consuming a fair amount tend to be affected less by caffeine.

Caffeine is a mildly addictive substance and people who consume large daily amounts can develop a dependency to it. Withdrawal may bring on the same symptoms that use of caffeine causes in others.

Are any of caffeine's effects harmful? In extreme cases, certainly. Caffeine can be fatal at doses of 10 grams ingested in 30 minutes. However, one cup of coffee has approximately 100 milligrams, so it is highly unlikely that coffee alone will provide deadly levels of caffeine. This would be 1,000 cups of strong coffee or 200 cans of cola. On the other hand, an overdose of some caffeine-containing medications could be fatal.

Americans are the second highest consumers of caffeine in the world (behind the Swedes). When all sources of caffeine are considered, 20 to 30 percent of American adults consume more than 500 milligrams of caffeine a day.

Caffeine is an ingredient in more than 1,000 nonprescription drug products as well as numerous prescription drugs. It is most often used in weight-control products, stay-awake tablets, headache and pain relief medicines, cold remedies, and diuretics. When caffeine is an ingredient it is listed on the product label. Some examples of caffeine-containing drugs are listed in the table on page 133.

Possible Harmful Effects of Caffeine

The FDA has advised pregnant women to avoid caffeine or use only small amounts of foods and drugs containing caffeine. Caffeine is a drug, and like most drugs, it enters the bloodstream and crosses the placental barrier to reach the fetus. The FDA warning was based on research in which birth defects were seen in offspring of rats force-fed exceedingly high amounts of caffeine. Although it isn't clear how the findings apply to humans, the FDA issued the warning because of widespread consumption of beverages, foods, and drugs containing caffeine.

In a more recent study, rats sipped varying levels of caffeine in their water throughout the day. In this study no birth defects were seen unless the pregnant rats had levels of caffeine equivalent to 18 or more cups of coffee per day.

In 1982, Harvard researchers published the results of a study on the effects of caffeine on the outcome of pregnancy in more than 12,000 women. They found no link between the amount of coffee consumed and birth defects. Additional U.S. and Finnish studies have arrived at the same conclusion.

However, to be on the safe side, pregnant women may still want to be cautious about consuming too many caffeine-containing foods and beverages, since caffeine does cross the placenta to the fetus.

Mothers who breast-feed are also warned about moderation in caffeine consumption. Actually, the few studies done on the transfer of caffeine from mothers to breast-fed infants have concluded that modest use of caffeinated beverages does not appear to present a hazard to the nursing infant. The possibility does exist, however, that frequent intake of large quantities of caffeine might cause it to accumulate in the baby, but to date there is no evidence to support this theory.

Other studies suggest that caffeine may be associated with a type of breast disease. Fibrocystic breast disease is a painful, noncancerous breast condition that occurs in approximately 10 to 20 percent of women. Some evidence suggests that removing from the diet all methyl xanthines, a group of chemicals which includes caffeine, may help control the development of these breast lumps. Methyl xanthines also include theophylline found in tea and theobromine found in chocolate.

Some researchers feel the studies of this breast disease are insufficient and the words of caution premature. A recent study involving 323 women with the disease and nearly 1,500 without it found no association between consumption of caffeine and other methyl xanthines and fibrocystic breast disease.

The debate over the possible association between heavy consumption of coffee and heart disease has continued for more than 30 years. The Framingham Heart Study found no association between coffee consumption and increased risk of heart problems. However, in a study investigating whether caffeine produces irregular heartbeats, it was found that the amount of caffeine contained in two cups of brewed coffee caused three heart patients to experience an increased heart rate and six other patients to have irregular heartbeats. Three healthy volunteers also had irregular heartbeats after receiving caffeine. The researchers concluded that caffeine has the potential to cause heartbeat irregularities, especially in patients with existing heart problems. They advised people who have heart problems to avoid caffeine.

A study conducted at Stanford University in 1985 has again drawn attention to caffeine. In a small group of men, it was found that those who drank more than 2 1/2 to 3 cups of coffee per day had higher average total cholesterol and LDL cholesterol levels. Normal cholesterol levels were found in men who drank less than 2 cups of coffee per day. However, the researchers noted the limitations of the study due to the small number of subjects and the subjects' similar backgrounds. They felt at this time that it was not possible to make a cause and effect conclusion which would be applicable to the general population.

Another study reported an increased risk of pancreatic cancer among coffee drinkers. But this study had a number of serious limitations and has been strongly criticized. Research in this area is very unclear and there is no definite answer.

Decaffeinated coffee has also come under close scrutiny because of the techniques used to remove caffeine from coffee beans. Until the mid-70s the most commonly used decaffeinator was trichloroethylene (TCE). Companies stopped using TCE in 1975 after the National Cancer Institute issued a warning that high doses of TCE had caused liver cancer in mice. Today companies use methylene chloride as a decaffeinator. Although the chemical has brief contact with the beans when it is applied and then roasted away, some people are concerned that the trace remaining might be harmful. However, scientists estimate that someone would have to consume huge amounts of decaffeinated coffee to experience any side-effects from the methylene chloride.

Many people have switched to herbal teas in hopes of avoiding caffeine. They may reduce caffeine intake but many herbal teas contain potent chemicals that alter normal functions of the body and mind. They can be a more serious health hazard than has ever been linked to caffeine.

Recommendations

As stated earlier, evidence seems to suggest that caffeine consumption in moderation is unlikely to pose a health risk for healthy people. Moderation is considered to be 3 cups or less of coffee or the equivalent amount of caffeine (250 milligrams) per day. However, drinking about 10 cups of coffee a day or daily consumption of more than 1,000 milligrams of caffeine in any form, may lead to caffeinism, or "coffee nerves."

Pregnant women and heart patients should probably be more careful about how much caffeine they consume. Persons on medications should check with their physician or pharmacist to see if taking caffeine along with their medications is a problem. Parents should be particularly careful about the amount of caffeine-containing foods and beverages their children consume.

If you decide to cut back on your caffeine intake, do it gradually. This will help prevent withdrawal symptoms. You may have experienced some of these withdrawal symptoms on weekends when your usual work "coffee breaks" are eliminated.

Tannin, the other ingredient of concern to coffee drinkers, is a bitter-tasting acid which increases as coffee brews, becoming overpowering if the coffee boils. To avoid excess tannin:

- Make sure never to boil coffee.
- Maintain the least possible time of contact between coffee and boiling water. This will also keep caffeine down to a minimum. The drip method is better than percolator-brewed coffee.
- Don't let perked coffee stand with coffee grounds.

The following list, compiled in 1983 by the Food and Drug Administration, shows the caffeine content of various soft drinks and foods.

CAFFEINE CONTENT OF BEVERAGES AND FOODS*

Item	Caffeine (milligrams) Average	Range
Coffee (5-oz. cup)		
Brewed, drip method	115	60-180
Brewed, percolator	80	40-170
Instant	65	30-120
Decaffeinated, brewed	3	2-5
Decaffeinated, instant	2	1-5
Tea (5-oz. cup)		
Brewed, major U.S. brands	40	20-90
Brewed, imported brands	60	25-110
Instant	30	25-50
Iced (12-oz. glass)	70	67-76
Cocoa and Chocolate		
Cocoa beverage (5-oz. cup)	4	2-20
Chocolate milk beverage (8 oz.)	5	2-7
Milk chocolate (1 oz.)	6	1-15
Dark chocolate, semi-sweet (1 oz.)	20	5-35
Baker's chocolate (1 oz.)	26	
Chocolate-flavored syrup (1 oz.)	4	
Soft drinks (12 oz.)		
Sugar-Free Mr. Pibb	59	
Mountain Dew	54	
Mello Yello	53	
Tab	47	
Coca-Cola	46	
Diet Coke	46	
Shasta Cola	45	
Shasta Cherry Cola	45	
Shasta Diet Cola	45	
Sunkist Orange	42	
Mr. Pibb	41	
Dr. Pepper	40	
Sugar-Free Dr. Pepper	40	
Pepsi Cola	38	
Diet Rite Cola	36	
RC Cola	36	
Pepsi Light	36	

Diet Pepsi	36
7-Up	0
RC-100	0
Fresca	0
Hires Root Beer	0

CAFFEINE CONTENT OF NONPRESCRIPTION DRUGS

Weight-Control Aids (daily dose)	
Codexin	200
Dex-A-Diet II	200
Dexatrim, Dexatrim Extra Strength	200
Dietac capsules	200
Maximum Strength Appedrine	100
Prolamine	140
Alertness Tablets	
Nodoz	100
Vivarin	200
Caffedrin Capsules	200
Analgesic/Pain Relief (standard dose)	
Anacin, Maximum Strength Anacin	32
Excedrin	65
Midol	32.4
Vanquish	33
Aspirin, plain (any brand)	0
Diuretics (standard dose)	
Aqua-Ban	100
Maximum Strength Aqua-Ban Plus	200
Permathene H_2 Off	200
Pre-Mens Forte	100
Cold/Allergy Remedies (standard dose)	
Coryban-D capsules	30
Triaminicin tablets	30
Dristan Decongestant tablets and Dristan A-F Decongestant tablets	16.2
Duradyne-Forte	30

*Source: FDA, Food Additive Chemistry Evaluation Branch and National Center for Drugs and Biologies, 1984.

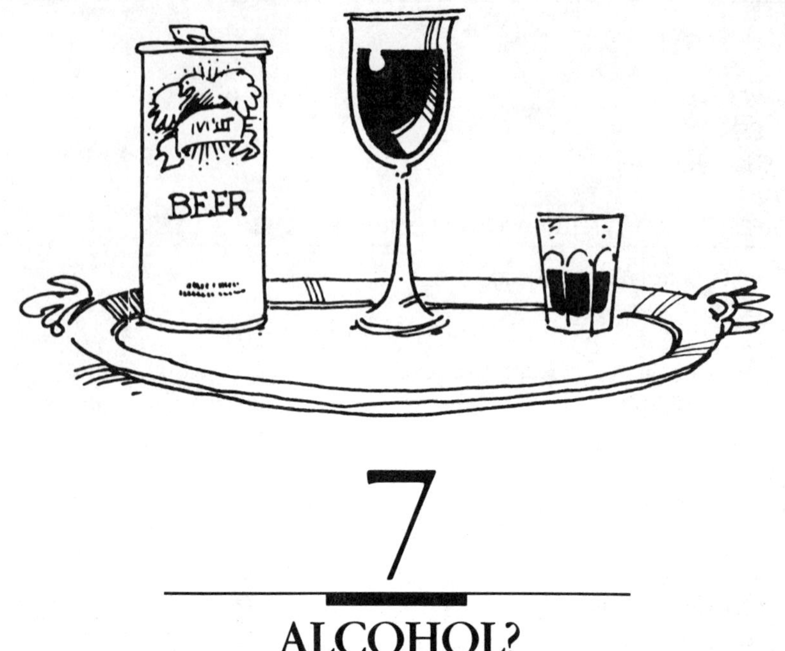

7

ALCOHOL?

An important nutritional key and overall healthy lifestyle factor is to keep an eye on alcohol consumption. Alcohol is high in calories and contains no vitamins and minerals. It is a toxic substance that depletes other nutrients in its metabolism (the process of breaking it down into compounds that can be used by the body). Besides being the primary factor in cirrhosis of the liver, alcohol has also been related to increased incidence of other maladies: cancer of the mouth, throat and esophagus; accidents; and birth defects.

Alcohol is unquestionably the nation's leading mood altering drug. We often think of alcohol as a stimulant, but actually alcohol has a depressant effect on the brain. The initial effect is to lift barriers of self-control, which is why alcohol appears to be a stimulant. However, as alcohol intake continues, it depresses brain function; coma and even death may follow. Fortunately, most drinkers rarely get beyond the relaxing effect of low levels of alcohol.

The average American consumes 210 calories a day in the form of alcohol. Wine consumption has risen to an average of 7 quarts yearly per person from 4 quarts 15 years ago. We now drink twice as much wine as orange juice!

Alcohol is absorbed from the stomach and the small intestine and goes directly to the liver. The liver can metabolize about an ounce of alcohol per hour. Amounts above that are circulated out into the general bloodstream to be returned later to the liver for metabolism. In this process of circulation, alcohol reaches the central nervous system and brain, causing the symptoms described above.

Because alcohol is a toxic substance, the liver metabolizes it before food and uses alcohol's calories as the body's source of energy. Calories from food that is eaten during this time will be converted to fat and stored in fatty tissue for future energy use. Alcohol calories not used immediately for energy are stored in the liver as fat. Years of heavy drinking can cause a "fatty liver" (accumulation of fat in the liver).

Alcoholic beverages can be high in calories. Pure alcohol contains 7 calories per gram. A half ounce of pure alcohol—the amount of alcohol in most one-ounce shots—contains approximately 80 to 90 calories. Along with calories from the alcohol, many alcoholic beverages also contain calories from carbohydrate in the sweeteners and mixers used with them.

Not only is alcohol itself a source of "empty calories," which means it gives the body fuel without any other nutrients, but it also deprives the body of nutrients from the foods we eat. Alcohol uses some vitamins in its metabolism and interferes with the absorption and storage of other vitamins.

"Proof" tells you the alcoholic content of distilled spirits (gin, bourbon, vodka, scotch, etc.). In the United States the proof value is equal to twice the percentage of alcohol by volume. One ounce of pure alcohol is 200 proof; 100 proof alcohol is 50 percent alcohol in each ounce (30 ml), or 15 grams of alcohol per ounce. The alcohol content of wine is given as a percentage; white wines are usually 12 percent and red wines 14 percent. Beer contains between 3 and 8 percent alcohol, with "light" beers usually containing the smaller amount. Liqueurs are usually 40 to 55 percent alcohol. A simple formula for calculating caloric content of alcohol beverages is:

$$0.8 \times \text{proof} \times \text{ounces} = \text{calories}$$

Some scientific studies have found that moderate alcohol intake is associated with an increased level of HDL (high density lipoprotein) cholesterol, which is the type of cholesterol that is protective against heart disease. This early finding led many to champion the moderate use of alcohol in the fight against heart disease! However, there are actually two classes of HDLs: HDL-2, which is the specific cholesterol associated with a reduction in coronary heart disease; and HDL-3, which is not related to heart disease. Further studies showed that moderate use of alcohol raised the HDL-3 level but not the HDL-2 level, and therefore it is not protective against heart disease. So it appears that the abstainers are winning out after all!

Problems With Large Doses

Alcohol is a factor in nearly half the nation's traffic fatalities as well as many other accidental deaths. This is a result of alcohol's dulling effect on the brain.

Since the liver is the body's means of detoxifying alcohol, prolonged heavy drinking can lead to liver damage. Spurts of heavy drinking can cause inflammation of the liver, which is called alcoholic hepatitis. Prolonged heavy drinking can lead to cirrhosis of the liver, a chronic and potentially fatal dysfunction of the liver that also increases risks of liver cancer.

Alcohol and smoking increase the risk of cancer. People who consume a lot of alcohol are far more likely to develop cancer of the mouth, throat, larynx, or esophagus. Alcohol can also damage the lining of the stomach and small intestine, interfering with the absorption of needed nutrients.

Although alcohol can stimulate an interest in sexual activity, it actually impairs sexual performance.

A special concern is the use of alcohol during pregnancy. In the mid-1970s researchers identified growth abnormalities and birth defects among babies of women who drank heavily during pregnancy. These problems are called fetal alcohol syndrome. They include malformation of facial characteristics, growth failure, and central nervous system problems resulting in a decrease in intellectual abilities and low IQ.

We know that when large amounts of alcohol are consumed, the alcohol leaves the liver and while in the bloodstream can cross the placenta to the fetus. Because the fetus is so small, it very quickly literally becomes drunk. Obviously you would not give alcohol to a small child, but it is even more important not to expose a developing fetus to alcohol.

It appears that even low doses of alcohol may result in growth failure and/or lower IQ. Moderate amounts of alcohol (1 ounce of pure alcohol taken twice a week) doubles the risk of spontaneous abortion as well as fetal growth failure. The most critical time for exposure to alcohol is very early in pregnancy. Unfortunately, this may be a time when the mother does not even realize she is pregnant.

As a result, pregnant women are being advised to limit alcohol intake to at most two drinks a day. Some experts suggest NO alcohol, but this is a decision that each woman must make. Alcohol is a drug which can and does affect the developing fetus. It is not known at this time if there is a level of daily alcohol consumption which is "safe" during pregnancy. As with alcohol, women should be extremely cautious about taking any kind of drug during pregnancy without first consulting their physician. Cigarette smoking can also cause infants of low birth weight.

Responsible Use of Alcohol

How much alcohol an individual can drink without becoming impaired or intoxicated depends on several factors, including body weight, food eaten, tiredness, and mental state. Prevention of alcoholic problems begins with the individual and the family practicing responsible attitudes and decisions about drinking.

The recommendation is to limit alcohol to less than five to six percent of the total calories per day, with no more than one to two ounces daily. One ounce of alcohol is defined as 1 1/2 ounces of 80 proof liquor such as gin, vodka, bourbon, whiskey or dry brandy; one 4-ounce glass of table wine; or one 12-ounce glass of beer.

Jane Brody, a medical writer for ***The New York Times***, in **Jane Brody's Nutrition Book**, lists the following general guidelines for responsible use of alcohol:

1. Eat something before and while you drink. Try to avoid salty snack foods that make you thirsty and increase the likelihood you will drink too much.
2. Lower the concentration of alcohol in your drink by diluting it with ice and a mixer.
3. Sip your drinks slowly.
4. Avoid situations in which drinking is the only "activity." Drink only in a relaxed, pleasant atmosphere.
5. Do not mix alcohol and other drugs and don't drink if taking medication. Alcohol dangerously increases the effects of many drugs and medications and can inactivate some medications.
6. Set limits to protect your dignity and self-respect.
7. Respect the abstainer.
8. Know your capacity and stick to it. The smaller you are the more you are likely to feel the effect of a given amount of alcohol. Research has also shown that women are generally more sensitive to alcohol than are men.
9. If you have overindulged in alcohol, only time will help you to sober up. In general it takes as many hours to recover as the number of drinks you have consumed.
10. If drinking, don't drive. Don't let an intoxicated friend get behind the wheel.
11. If alcohol is a problem, get help.

If you are hosting a party, help your guests by:

1. Respecting abstainers by providing attractive choices for them as well. Hot or cold punch drinks can be an attractive alternative to alcoholic drinks. On warm summer days, serve frosty tall glasses of punch that is colorful and refreshing. On chilly winter days, a steaming cup of something hot warms the body and the heart.

   Punch loses its "punch" if not served very cold or very hot. When serving cold punch, chill all ingredients before mixing in a non-metallic container. Add carbonated beverages just before serving, and mix only to blend, so carbonation is not lost. For hot punches, make sure the punch bowl is heat resistant before adding hot punch. It will help to warm the bowl with hot water before adding the punch.

2. Offering lower alcohol and lower calorie drinks. Fruit juices give you vitamins and minerals; alcohol gives you only calories. A 6-ounce glass of fruit juice averages 95 calories and a 6-ounce glass of tomato juice has 35 calories. Both are better choices than alcohol. Spritzers (half wine and half club soda) can be an excellent way to dilute alcohol and are available at most bars.

3. Not making drinks too strong and not forcing refills of alcoholic drinks on your guests.

4. Providing food along with beverages. Snacks that are too salty increase thirst, so try other healthy food choices.

The table on the next page lists the caloric content of some alcoholic drinks:

CALORIC CONTENT OF ALCOHOLIC BEVERAGES

	Serving Size (oz.)	Calories Per Serving	Calories From Alcohol
Beer			
Regular beer	12	150-175	93-123
Light beer	12	95	82
Extra light beer	12	70	57
Near beer	12	65	9
Liquor—Jigger =1½ oz.			
Gin, Rum, Vodka, Whiskey (86 proof)	1½	105	105
Dry Brandy or Cognac	1	75	75
Wine			
Red or Rosé	3½	85	81
Sweet	3½	102	83
Dry white	3½	80	79
Light wine	3½	50	45
Champagne	4	98	83
Sweet Kosher	4	132	83
Sherry	2	73	65
Sweet sherry, port, muscatel	2	94	65
Vermouth			
Dry	3	105	88
Sweet	3	141	85
Mixed Drinks			
Ingredients and proportions vary, but most mixed drinks are about 4 ounces and 200 calories.			
Cocktails			
Bloody Mary	10	264	210
Daiquiri	4	139	120
Eggnog	4	370	140
Gin & Tonic	10	212	140
Gin Rickey	4	150	147
Mai Tai	4	258	244
Manhatten	4	187	152

continued

	Serving Size (oz.)	Calories Per Serving	Calories From Alcohol
Margarita	4	254	218
Martini	4	250	249
Old Fashioned	4	179	168
Planters Punch	4	200	176
Screwdriver	8	232	140
Tom Collins (w/o mix)	10	173	140
Tom Collins (with mix)	10	252	140
Liqueurs			
Anisette Cordial	2/3	74	49
Benedictine	2/3	69	49
Creme de menthe	2/3	67	49
Curacao	2/3	54	42
General (fruit, chocolate coffee)	2/3	70-115 (avg. 66)	42
Cocktail Mixes			
Club soda	8	0	
Cola	8	96	
Ginger ale	8	72	
Mineral water	8	0	
Quinine water (tonic)	8	72	
Seltzer	8	0	
Tom Collins mixes	8	112	

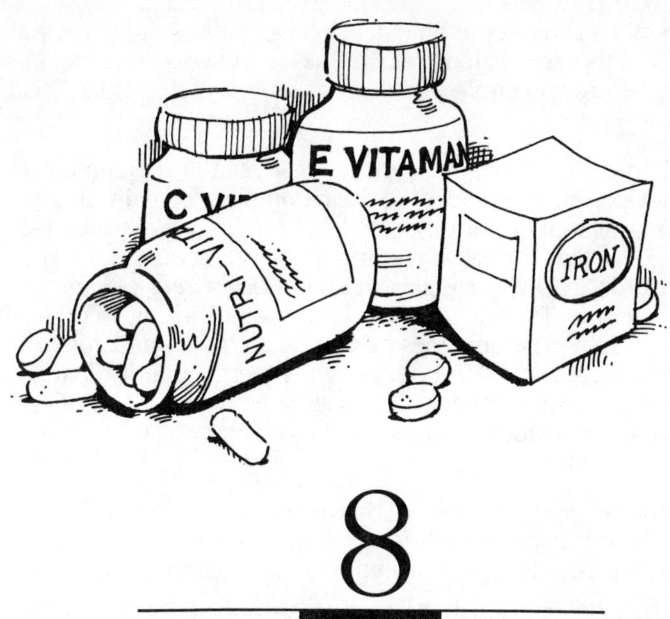

8

VITAMINS AND MINERALS: TO SUPPLEMENT OR NOT TO SUPPLEMENT?

The advertisement shows a person who watches his or her diet, gets plenty of exercise, and "just to be sure," takes a vitamin and mineral supplement every day. The implication of such advertising has contributed to the myth that even a balanced diet cannot provide adequate nutrients.

Should vitamin or mineral supplements be used? For hundreds of thousands of years, people got all the vitamins and minerals they needed from the food they ate. But now many people feel our modern lifestyles have gotten them into nutritional trouble. Processed foods, drugs, cigarettes, and alcohol can interfere with adequate nutrition. People who rely on a limited number or type of foods are the most susceptible to a nutritionally inadequate diet. However, for most people, increasing consumption of common foods rich in certain vitamins will more than provide adequate nutrition.

There are certain individuals who can benefit from a multivitamin supplement. Infants are commonly given vitamin supplements, as are pregnant women and nursing mothers. Others likely to fall short of essential vitamins are heavy smokers, women on oral contraceptives, heavy drinkers, users of certain drugs, surgical and other ill patients, elderly persons and people on extended weight loss programs with very major cutbacks in caloric intake. Ask a dietitian, doctor, or nurse for advice before you take extra vitamins for any of the above situations.

If you fall into one of these categories, your vitamin supplement should not exceed 100 percent of the recommended daily allowance (RDA) for a vitamin or mineral. The label on the bottle, which lists percentages of RDA for each vitamin, can serve as your guide. The RDA standards are set up to meet the nutritional needs of large groups of people. They are not standards for individuals. Because they must cover many different types of people, the RDA standards include a generous safety factor. Most people will meet their individual needs by including two-thirds of an RDA for any one nutrient. The RDA includes those individuals who for some reason need more of a particular nutrient.

It makes no difference to your body whether you take so-called "natural" vitamins or those made in laboratories. Two major fallacies lie behind the rush for the so-called "natural" vitamin:

1. The false belief that natural vitamins are superior to those made by man (synthesized).
2. The false belief that vitamin products sold as "natural" don't contain synthetic ingredients.

In truth, each vitamin has a particular molecular structure that remains the same whether it is made in a laboratory or taken from an animal or plant. The body cannot distinguish between a natural and a synthetic form of a given chemical.

While there is no difference in the basic form of vitamins and minerals, there can be a large difference in the amount and balance in which they occur naturally in foods versus when they are taken as supplements. The best way to get your daily requirement of essential vitamins and minerals is through the foods you eat. This way you won't distort the proper balance and amounts of the various vitamins and minerals. By choosing carefully from a wide variety of foods and by preparing and storing those foods properly, you can do a great deal to protect the nutritional value of the foods you eat.

An inadequate intake of any nutrient can result in a deficiency problem, while too much of some nutrients can result in toxicity. Doses at which toxic effects may occur have been identified for most vitamins, including vitamins A and C, which are popular among nonprescription users. Toxic effects are most likely with fat-soluble vitamins, which can build up over time in the fatty tissue of the body.

Fat-Soluble Vitamins: A, D, E, K

Water-Soluble Vitamins: Vitamin C and the B vitamins—thiamine, riboflavin, niacin, folacin, B6, B12, biotin

Little is known of possible long-term hazards associated with the taking of high doses of vitamins over long periods of time. People who take megadose quantities of nutrients are no longer taking vitamins, they are taking drugs. Even some of the water-soluble B vitamins, which are commonly thought to be non-toxic because they are cleared from the body in the urine, are now known to cause serious problems in megadose quantities (10 or more times the RDA).

Although excessive amounts of water-soluble vitamins are excreted in the urine, they can cause problems while passing through the body. A study has shown that vitamin B6 (pyridoxine) megadoses can cause severe neurological problems including numbness, difficulty walking, sharp pain, and loss of normal reflexes. These symptoms went away after megadoses of this vitamin were stopped, but often recovery took more than a year.

Folic acid supplements taken in large doses can mask symptoms of vitamin B deficiency. Niacin megadoses cause flushing of the face, neck and chest; abnormal heart rhythms, itching, headaches, cramps, nausea and vomiting, diarrhea, abnormally low blood pressure, fast heartbeat, and dry skin.

Vitamin C megadoses can cause mild diarrhea and abdominal cramps and may cause formation of kidney stones. If megadoses are abruptly stopped, scurvy can result. Infants of mothers using megadoses of vitamin C during pregnancy have also been shown to develop symptoms of scurvy when they no longer have that large amount.

Excessive amounts of the fat-soluble vitamins A, D, E, and K are especially dangerous. These vitamins are stored in the body in fatty tissue and can accumulate to toxic levels if excessive doses are taken. Vitamin A has been the cause of the largest number of cases of vitamin poisoning. Its unproved association with cancer prevention has been partly responsible for this.

All of our vitamins, minerals, and other nutrients work together in a balanced manner and it is important not to distort this balance. As an example, proper calcium metabolism is dependent on the presence of the right amounts of protein, phosphorus, vitamin D, fat and fiber.

In summary:

1. Eat a balanced diet which contains items from the four major food groups. If you are worried that your diet does not contain enough of the needed nutrients, write down everything you eat

for seven days and have it analyzed by a registered dietitian. She/he can tell you if your food choices are appropriate, and if they are not, can advise you on how to improve the nutritional value of your diet by changing your food choices.

2. Learn to purchase, store, and prepare food in ways that enhance and preserve the vitamins.

3. If you decide to use a supplement in addition to a balanced diet, use a multivitamin supplement which contains no more than 100% of the RDA for each vitamin and mineral.

4. If you purchase a supplement, remember that many of the synthetic brands are just as good as the more expensive "natural" brands.

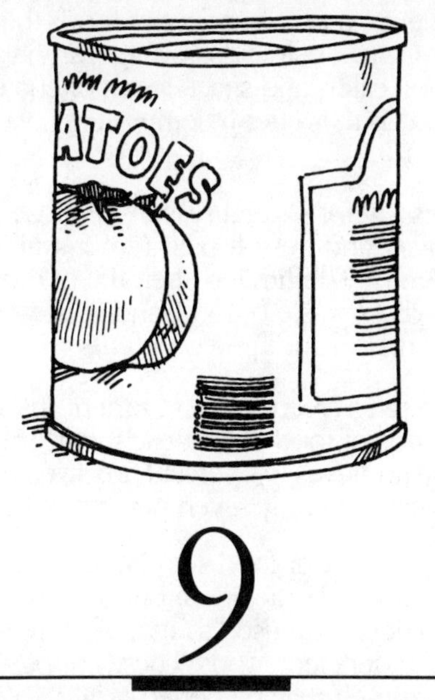

9

CONCERNS ABOUT FOOD ADDITIVES

The food label reads:

> water, starches, cellulose, pectin, fructose, sucrose, glucose, malic acid, citric acid, succinic acid, anisyl propionate, amyl acetate, ascorbic acid, beta carotene, riboflavin, thiamin, niacin, phosphorus, and potassium.

Is this a healthy food for a nutrition-conscious consumer? Absolutely! As is pointed out in **Jane Brody's Nutrition Book**, the label is for cantaloupe, a low-calorie food rich in vitamins.

The point is, all food is made up of chemicals. Not all chemicals are bad, whether they're natural or manufactured in the laboratory. Neither are all chemicals good.

Should we become overly concerned about food additives? There are currently 1,300 food additives approved for use as colors, flavors, preservatives, thickeners and other agents for controlling the physical properties of food. These additives serve a wide variety of purposes. They make possible many safe and nutritious convenience foods, such as packaged breads, canned fruits and vegetables, margarine and ready-to-eat cereals.

Additives are, however, most abundant in foods that we would be better off without. Candy, cold cuts, sausage, artificial or sugary beverages, packaged cakes and snack foods often contain many additives. All are foods that offer little nutritional value or contain too much fat, sugar or salt.

Additives are necessary for several reasons. Foods spoil quickly without preservatives, and fresh foods are not available all year or in all parts of the country. The limited shelf life of most fresh foods would lead to needless waste of food, and food would cost more because of transportation and time problems.

Additives make up ten percent of most Americans' diets. Of the average 1,500 pounds of food we eat each year, 150 pounds are additives. Of those additives, 93 percent are sweeteners and salt. Other chemicals make up only seven percent of the total.

Food additives that keep our food supply safe to eat have a valid purpose and can't always be avoided. But other additives simply improve marketability or are used to manufacture synthetic, high-calorie, nutritionally deficient foods. These are best avoided, even though the additive itself may be perfectly safe.

To help reduce your exposure to needless additives:*

- Eat a variety of foods to help dilute the concentration of additives in any one food and to minimize the chances that a single additive will reach unsafe levels in your body.
- Use fresh or minimally processed foods.
- Use "real foods," not their artificial equivalents.
- Pay attention to food labels when you shop.
- Don't be fooled by the word "natural" on the label. "All natural" does not mean additive-free, since many additives are natural substances.
- Don't forget the two leading additives—sugar and salt.

*Adapted from **Jane Brody's Nutrition Book**.

10

PUTTING IT ALL TOGETHER

The final key to putting together all the specific nutritional keys for opening the door to good nutrition is to make changes you enjoy. Remember that food habits are formed from infancy. Your individual tastes are a result of a lifetime of learned experiences with food. Don't try to change all your eating habits at once. Develop an Eating Management Plan based on small, step-by-step changes, and discover foods that allow you to enjoy your new way of eating.

You may feel you need professional help to assist you in the planning and implementation of changes you feel are important. The professional who can help you is a Registered Dietitian (R.D.). An R.D. can help you plan an appropriate caloric level and meal plan which will meet the goal of a nutritionally healthy food intake with which you feel comfortable.

Many R.D.s use a meal planning system based on exchange lists of foods. This is a system of grouping foods according to calories and nutrient content. There are six exchange lists: milk, vegetable, fruit, bread (starch), meat, and fat. Meals and snacks for each day (a meal plan) are based on a specific number of servings from each exchange list. Using this system, a meal plan can be individualized to meet nutritional goals.

Start by assessing your current food intake patterns. An R.D. can also help you do this. Then determine small, realistic goals for change in each food group to achieve a healthier eating style. Work toward the specific goals by making small step-by-step changes. Begin by making changes in your fat and sugar intake. These changes will also help you reach your desirable body weight. Then make changes to increase complex carbohydrate and reduce salt and alcohol. You will notice that this book is arranged in approximately that order. Remember that gradual changes have the best chance of becoming part of your lifestyle.

Your attitude is an important part of your Eating Management Plan. You need to:

1. ***Be Realistic:*** To set goals that are too high or unrealistic is to set the stage for failure. Remember to plan changes in small, gradual steps.

2. ***Be Flexible:*** The key is to make lasting food selection changes you can enjoy. If you find you can't enjoy one food, look for an equally healthy alternative.

3. ***Develop A Problem-Solving Attitude:*** If you find a particular food or habit is hard to change, learn to turn that difficulty into an opportunity to solve a problem. As an example, when you have ice cream in your home freezer, you may find it difficult to resist large servings daily. By thinking through the problem, you may decide it is unrealistic to completely avoid ice cream, but by not purchasing it for your home freezer, you can keep ice cream as a "treat" when eating out or for special occasions.

4. ***Use Positive Self-Dialogue:*** Self-dialogues (internal conversations) play an important part in evaluating your self-management efforts. What you say to yourself makes a difference in the way you behave and the way you feel. So think positive thoughts about positive actions.

We've introduced you to some of the most important guidelines for good nutrition. Following the specific recommendations discussed in previous chapters should result in an adventure in good eating and a healthier lifestyle. By enjoying the changes you make, you can successfully maintain them for a lifetime.

The rest of this book will focus on guidelines related to food purchasing, food preparation, meal planning, and eating away from home.

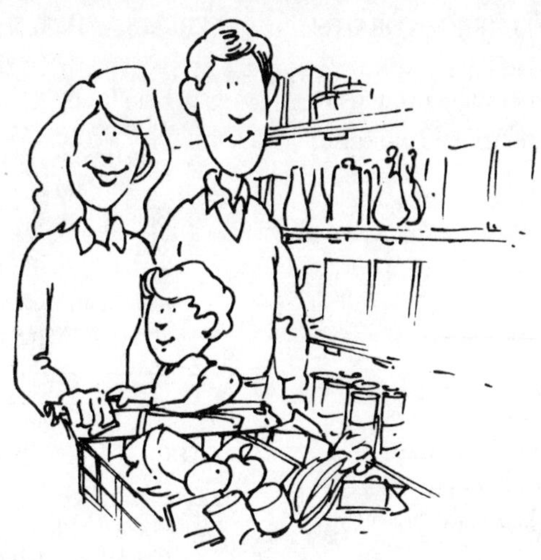

Food Purchasing

One of the first ways to change food choices is to change the foods you bring into your home. Food purchasing suggestions have been listed under specific food areas in this book. Some general recommendations for food purchasing are:

- Plan ahead. Remember that this is the key to wise food purchasing. What you purchase on that weekly grocery trip will determine your food choices throughout the week.
- Outline your weekly menu, taking into consideration new recipes or foods you want to try that will help you achieve your specific nutritional goals.
- Plan your grocery list from your menu and from those food choices you will want on hand for making eating changes.
- Be sure to make your grocery trip when your stomach is full. You are more likely to shop carelessly and stray from your grocery list when you are hungry. See sample grocery list on pages 150-151.
- Try to buy just those items on the list. The list should be complete enough so that daily trips to the store can be avoided.
- Avoid buying foods you tend to overeat, especially those high calorie foods. Spend more time in the produce section when looking for snacking items to "have around the house."
- Be wary of attractive displays and tempting advertising techniques that make you buy without thinking.
- Learn to read labels and become product-wise.

TEAM UP WITH CARBOHYDRATES!

FRUITS — High in fiber
— High in vitamin A and C

All fresh, frozen, or canned, no sugar added

___ Grapes
___ Oranges
___ Grapefruit
___ Strawberry
___ Bananas
___ Apples
___ Canteloupe
___ Watermelon
___ ____________________
___ ____________________

All juices fresh, frozen or canned, no sugar added

___ ____________________
___ ____________________

VEGETABLES — High in fiber
— Low in sodium
— High in Vitamin A and C

All fresh, frozen vegetables

___ Broccoli
___ Celery
___ Cabbage
___ Lettuce
___ Squash
___ Cucumbers
___ Peppers
___ Carrots
___ ____________________
___ ____________________
___ ____________________

BREADS — High fiber

Whole Grain Bread (first ingredient)

___ Stone ground
___ Whole wheat flour
___ Cracked wheat
___ English muffin
___ Bagels
___ Tortillas — corn or whole wheat
___ ____________________
___ ____________________
___ ____________________

CEREALS — High fiber
— Less sugar

___ Bran Buds
___ All Bran
___ 40% Bran Flakes
___ Raisin Bran
___ Bran Chex
___ Total
___ Wheaties
___ Nutrigrain — rye, wheat, corn
___ Shredded Wheat
___ ____________________
___ ____________________

OTHER — High fiber

___ Brown rice
___ Potato, white
___ Crackers — whole wheat, low salt
___ Graham Crackers
___ Popcorn
___ Dried beans and peas (pinto, lima, navy, lentils, kidney)
___ Whole wheat flour
___ Pasta and noodles
___ Bulgur
___ ____________________
___ ____________________
___ ____________________

LEAN TOWARD LEAN!

MEAT, FISH, POULTRY — Low in fat

___ Beef
___ Ground (lean)
___ Chuck
___ Flank steak
___ Tenderloin
___ Top round
___ Bottom round
___ Rump
___ Round
___ ____________________
___ Veal
___ ____________________
___ Chicken
___ ____________________
___ Turkey
___ ____________________
___ Fish (without breading or sauce)
___ ____________________
___ ____________________

___ Tuna Fish (water packed)
___ Pork
___ ____________________
___ ____________________
___ Liver
___ ____________________
___ ____________________

CHEESE — High in calcium
— Low in fat
— Low in sodium

___ Farmers
___ Feta
___ Mozzarella — skim milk
___ Neufchatel (lowfat cream cheese)
___ Ricotta — skim milk
___ Parmesan
___ Cottage cheese — (2% or 4%)

MILK — High in calcium
— Low in fat

___ Ice milk
___ Low fat milk — 1 to 2%
___ Skim milk
___ Lowfat yogurt — plain
___ ____________________

FATS & OILS — Polyunsaturated oils

___ Margarines (liquid oil first ingredient)
___ Polyunsaturated vegetable oil (corn, safflower, soybean, sunflower)
___ Salad dressings made with polyunsaturated oils as first ingredient
___ Salad dressing mixes made with oil, water, vinegar, lowfat yogurt, mayonnaise, or buttermilk
___ Pam — cooking spray
___ Mayonnaise
___ Diet margarine
___ Diet mayonnaise
___ ____________________

SHAKE THE SALT HABIT!

MISCELLANEOUS

___ No salt tomato paste
___ No salt canned tomatoes
___ No salt mustard
___ No salt catsup
___ Spice blends (Mrs. Dash)
___ Adolf Natural Meat Tenderizer (low sodium)
___ Spices — powdered without salt
___ No salt potato or corn chips
___ Fresh herbs
___ ____________________
___ ____________________

Adapted from: Scott and White Clinic's Options Programs

Label Reading

Reading and understanding food labels can help you make wise food choices. An important part of the food label is the list of ingredients. Ingredients are listed in descending order of amounts; that is, the main ingredient is listed first and the smallest ingredient last. As you check the ingredients list of a product, note:

1. The order of the ingredients.
2. Ingredients to limit or avoid. Be aware of other names for fat, sugar and salt.

Listed below are ingredients you may wish to limit or avoid, followed on the next page with a list of generally acceptable ingredients:

INGREDIENTS TO LIMIT OR AVOID

High Saturated Fat Ingredients:

animal fat	lamb fat
bacon fat	lard
beef fat	meat fat
butter	milk chocolates
chicken fat	palm or palm kernel oil
cocoa butter	pork fat
coconut	shortening
coconut oil	turkey fat
cream and cream sauces	vegetable fat*
egg and egg yolk solids	vegetable oil*
hardened fat or oil	vegetable shortening
hydrogenated fat or oil	whole milk solids

*Usually palm or coconut oil

High Sodium Ingredients:

salt (sodium chloride)	bouillon
monosodium glutamate	baking powder
brine (salt and water)	soy sauce
broth	

Sources of Sugar:

sucrose	honey
fructose	molasses
dextrose	maple syrup
corn syrup	brown sugar
invert sugar	

ACCEPTABLE INGREDIENTS	
carob powder	monoglycerides
cocoa	nonfat dry milk or solids
corn oil	safflower oil
cottonseed oil	sesame oil
diglycerides	soybean oil, partially hydrogenated
hydrolyzed ingredients	
sunflower oil	

In addition to the list of ingredients, many food labels provide nutritional labeling or "nutrition information per serving." This information also can be of help to you in controlling fat, sodium, and sugar intake. Here is an example:

NUTRITION INFORMATION
(per serving)

Serving Size = 1 cup

Servings per container = 2

Calories	110
Protein	1 Gram
Carbohydrate	25 Grams
Fat	1 Gram
Sodium	275 Milligrams (970 mg/100 gm)

Percentage of U.S. Recommended Daily Allowances (U.S. RDA)

Protein	2
Vitamin A	25
Vitamin C	25
Thiamine	25
Riboflavin	25
Niacin	25
Calcium	4
Iron	4

Manufacturers making any nutritional claim for their products must by law include the following information:

1. ***Serving size***—the amount of food for which nutrition information is given, such as 1 slice, 1 cup or 3 ounces. The number of servings per container is also given.
2. ***Food energy***—the total number of calories and amounts of protein, fat, and carbohydrate (in grams) furnished by one serving of the food as it comes from the container. One gram of carbohydrate or protein supplies four calories, and one gram of fat supplies nine calories.
3. ***Percentage of the U.S. Recommended Daily Allowances (U.S. RDA)***—the protein, vitamin A, vitamin C, three B vitamins (thiamine, niacin, riboflavin), calcium, and iron in percentages furnished by a serving of the food as it comes from the container.
4. ***Other nutrient information***—the amounts of cholesterol or saturated and polyunsaturated fat are included if a nutritional claim is made; for example, "low-fat product."
5. ***Sodium content***—Listing the milligrams of sodium in the serving size or per 100 milligrams is required as of July 1986 on products bearing nutrition labels. Foods that do not carry a nutrition label are exempt from this rule. The label regulations for sodium claims were discussed in Chapter 5.

Other food labeling regulations to be aware of include:

- ***Low calorie:*** Food must contain no more than 40 calories per serving, but a food naturally low in calories cannot be so labeled.
- ***Reduced calories:*** must be at least one-third lower in calories than the food it is replacing. In addition, a comparison must be made to show what the "reduced calorie" claim is based on.
- ***Imitation:*** synthetic food products made to resemble natural foods but which are not nutritionally equal. This does not necessarily mean that they will not be acceptable or useful food products. For example, the product may be lower in fat than the product it is replacing. It would have to be labeled "imitation" but may be better to use than the original food product.

Following the nutritional guidelines as you purchase food will help you eat better—and save money. The most dramatic savings occur when sugars are decreased; soft drinks, candy, sweet baked goods and pre-sweetened cereals are expensive items. Lean cuts of beef, chicken and turkey are usually less expensive than prime beef, lamb, and many processed meats. Margarine is less expensive than butter. Reducing the amounts of salad dressing, catsup and sauces can also cut expenses. Home prepared foods also are less expensive than convenience foods, and unprocessed grain products cost less than refined grains.

Food Preparation

Once the food is home, you can prepare it in a way that decreases the amounts of fat, sugar, calories and salt. In the same way that you slowly make food changes, make your food preparation changes in small steps. Here is a good sequence:

1. **Begin with new cooking methods for common foods.** Learn to broil, boil, steam, bake, etc., instead of frying.
2. **Use recipe modification techniques.** Recipe modifications allow you to reduce the amount of fat, sugar and salt in a recipe. See the following section.
3. **Try new recipes and food products.** You might want to experiment. Before you launch your efforts, gather some cookbooks that will help you make a more pleasurable transition to healthier eating. See the list of Recommended Books on page 176.

How To Modify Recipes

You can modify recipes to reduce calories, total fat, saturated fat, cholesterol, sodium and/or concentrated sweets. The two basic ways to modify a recipe are to change a cooking technique or to change an ingredient. An example of changing a cooking technique would be to saute vegetables in broth instead of oil or butter, thus reducing total fat as well as possibly the type of fat. You can modify ingredients by reducing them, eliminating them completely, or by substituting a more acceptable ingredient.

To reduce an ingredient, analyze the function of the ingredient in a recipe. Is it a necessary part of the final product, such as sugar in a cake? If so, you may not be able to eliminate the ingredient completely. But you may be able to reduce the amount used. Products that can be eliminated are those added for appearance or because of habit and tradition. These products may be high in sodium or sugar.

Many substitutions can be made in recipes to lower the fat and cholesterol content. While taste and texture may change, the results are often just as pleasing. Remember—"The proof of the pudding is in the eating."

Possible substitutions to consider are:

- ***Evaporated skim milk for cream.*** However, in order to whip evaporated skim milk it must be partially frozen.
- ***Skim milk for whole milk.***
- ***Egg substitutes for whole eggs.*** However, some egg substitutes may have objectionable flavors. Flavor extracts may help disguise

them. Using two egg whites in place of one egg is another possibility.

- ***Margarine for butter.*** However, soft or tub margarines will not cream. Diet margarines contain more water and less fat and cannot be substituted ounce per ounce for butter.
- ***Oils for hydrogenated fats (shortening).*** However, crusts may not have the same flakiness, and dough may stick to rolling pins. Oils will not cream. One cup of shortening can be replaced by 3/4 cup of oil; 1/2 cup shortening by 1/3 cup of oil.
- ***Cocoa plus oil for chocolate.*** However, cocoa will not solidify to form a coating.
- ***Whole grains for refined ones.***
- ***In addition, you can reduce or eliminate salt in recipes.*** However, when you eliminate salt, breads may not rise at the same rate. But pasta and vegetables will cook in unsalted water just as well as in salted water.

Consider the following recipe modifications:

RECIPE MODIFICATIONS FOR LOWERING FAT AND REFINED CARBOHYDRATES

For	Try
1 whole egg	1/4 cup egg substitute or 1 egg white + 1 tsp. vegetable oil or 2 egg whites
1 cup butter	1 cup margarine
1 cup shortening or lard	3/4 cup vegetable oil
1/2 cup shortening	1/3 cup vegetable oil
1 cup whole milk	1 cup skim milk
1 cup light cream	1 cup evaporated skim milk or 3 Tbsp. oil and skim milk to equal 1 cup
1 cup heavy cream	1 cup evaporated skim milk or 2/3 cup skim milk and 1/3 cup oil
1 cup sour cream	1 cup plain yogurt or 1 cup blenderized low-fat cottage cheese (with lemon juice)
1 ounce regular cheese	1 oz. low calorie or skim milk cheese

continued

For	Try
2 Tbsp. flour (as thickener)	1 Tbsp. cornstarch
1 Tbsp. salad dressing	1 Tbsp. low-calorie salad dressing
1 oz. (1 square) baking chocolate	3 Tbsp. powdered cocoa and 1 Tbsp. oil
1 can condensed soup	Homemade skim milk white sauce (see page 65)
cream of celery	1 cup sauce + 1/4 cup chopped celery
cream of chicken	1¼ cup sauce + 1 chicken bouillon
cream of mushroom	1 cup sauce + 1 can drained mushrooms
Cream cheese	Blend 4 Tbsp. margarine with 1 cup dry low-fat cottage cheese. Salt to taste; small amount of skim milk is needed in blending.
1 oz. bacon (2 strips)	1 oz. lean Canadian bacon or 1 oz. lean ham
1 cup all-purpose white flour	1 cup whole wheat flour minus 2 Tbsp.; also, decrease the amount of oil called for in the recipe by 1 Tbsp. and increase the liquid called for by 1-2 Tbsp.; or use 1/2 cup white + 1/2 cup whole wheat flour; or use 3/4 cup white and 1/4 cup wheat germ and/or bran
White rice	Brown rice
Sugar	Reduce amount. Reduction can be up to 1/2 of the original amount. Use no more than 1/4 cup of added sweetener (sugar, honey, molasses, etc.) per cup of flour.
Fat	Use no more than 1/2 Tbsp. of added oil or fat per cup of flour; compensate by increasing low-fat moisture ingredient, such as buttermilk, to add moistness.
Salt	Reduce amount, try spices and herbs.

EXAMPLE OF RECIPE MODIFICATION*

Unmodified Beef Stroganoff

Ingredients:

1½ pounds lean beef
3 Tbsp. butter
3/4 Tbsp. finely chopped onion
3/4 pound sliced mushrooms
Salt, pepper, nutmeg
1/2 tsp. basil
1/4 cup white wine
1 cup cream or cultured sour cream cream

YIELD: Serves 4

Nutrients Per Serving:

Calories	536
Protein	38 grams
Total Fat	39 grams
Total Carbohydrate	6 grams
Cholesterol	172 mg.

Modified Beef Stroganoff

Ingredients:

1 pound lean beef
2 Tbsp. margarine
3/4 Tbsp. finely chopped onion
1 pound sliced mushrooms
Salt, pepper, nutmeg
1/2 tsp. basil
1/4 cup white wine
1 cup plain low-fat yogurt

YIELD: Serves 4

Nutrients Per Serving:

Calories	263
Protein	30 grams
Total Fat	12 grams
Total Carbohydrate	8 grams
Cholesterol	76 mg.

*Adapted from MRFIT Minneapolis Clinical Center Nutrition Educational Materials.

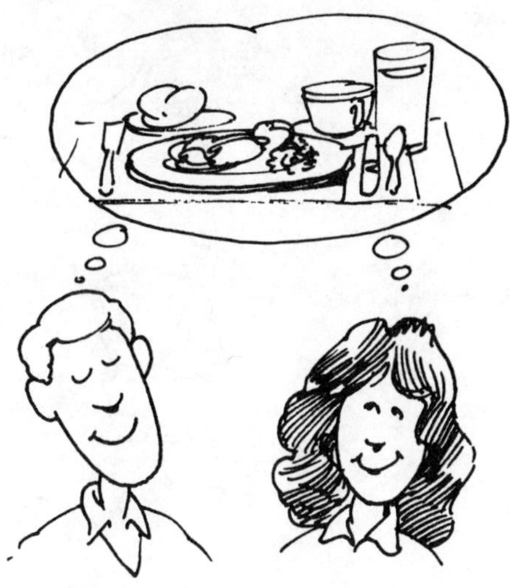

Meal Planning

Menu planning is an important skill. Our changing, fast-paced lifestyles often require foods which can be prepared quickly, yet are still nutritious and satisfying.

In menu planning, you need to consider how overall nutritional needs will fit into your meal plan. Also think about variety in color, taste and texture; time of year and food availability; preparation time; and total day's menus. When planning individual meals, follow these guidelines:

1. Begin by selecting the entree for the meal. Be imaginative and think of entrees that are not entirely meat dominated.
2. Next, plan the accompaniments to the entree—starch, vegetable, fruit.
3. Select appetizer, beverages and dessert (if desired).
4. Always include variety in menus—in flavor, color, temperature and texture. Flavors should blend together, not compete with each other. A creative menu is cohesive but has variety.
5. Choose garnishes and serving pieces for an attractive table setting.
6. The best choices for desserts are fresh fruit and fruit canned without sugar (in its own juice), sherbet, fruit whip, angel food cake, cakes or desserts made with appropriate ingredients (cocoa, unflavored gelatin, etc.). Decrease choices from cream products, fried foods, chocolate puddings and desserts, coconut, most commercial cakes, pies, cookies and mixes.

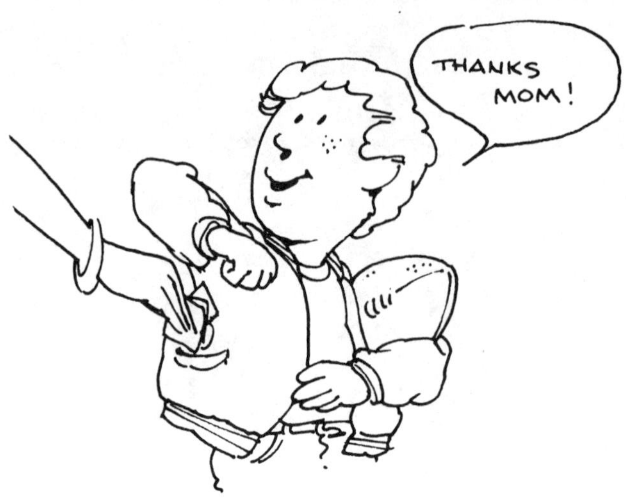

Planning for Snacks

Many commercial snacks are made with animal fats or hydrogenated vegetable fats and are high in sodium. They contribute a significant amount of fat, salt and calories to the diets of many people. You may want to assess the role these snacks play in your diet and look for alternatives.

Sale of salty snacks is a $6.1 billion dollar industry. The average American household consumes 28.6 pounds of salty snacks per year. Of this amount, 44.1% is potato chips, 24.1% corn tortilla chips, 14.9% salted nuts, 5.2% salted meat snacks, 4.8% pretzels, 4.6% other salted snacks, and 2.3% popped popcorn.

The following are hints for choosing snack foods:

- Buy or prepare snacks that are low in sodium and fat. If high sodium and fatty snacks are not in the house, they will be hard to eat.
- When you have time to prepare your own snacks, modify your recipes. Cut down the amount of sugar and use skim milk, margarine, oils, egg whites or egg substitutes.
- When preparing other snacks, try seasoning with spices such as basil, dill, lemon juice and garlic or onion powder instead of salt. Use fruit juices as a sweetener.
- Keep fruits and vegetables on hand in the refrigerator to satisfy those munchy moods.
- If you are trying to lose weight, avoid nuts, seeds, dried fruits and modified sweets that may be ***healthful*** but not necessarily ***helpful*** in reducing calories.

SODIUM, FAT, AND CALORIC CONTENT OF TYPICAL SNACK FOODS

Calories Per Serving	Serving Size	Sodium (milligrams)	Fat (grams)	Calories
Candy:				
Hershey's Chocolate Bar	1.4 oz.	35	13	220
Reese's Peanut Butter Cup-2 cups	1.8 oz.	110	14	270
Krackel Bar	1.4 oz.	40	12	210
Cakes (Snack):				
Hostess Ding Dong	1	96	9	170
Hostess Suzy Q	1	137	10	230
Hostess Twinkie	1	241	5	145
Chips: Frito's Corn Chips	1 oz.	204	10	160
Mister Salty Pretzel Sticks	1 oz.	830	1	120
Lay's Potato Chips	1 oz.	188	11	160
Doritos Tortilla Chips	1 oz.	193	7	142
Cookies:				
Nabisco Fig Newtons	2	125	2	120
Nabisco Oreos	3	200	7	155
Nabisco Nutter Butter	2	135	6	140
Crackers:				
Nabisco Ritz	4	125	3	70
Nabisco Wheat Thins	8	125	3	70
Nabisco Cheese Nips	13	195	3	70

Alternative Snack Choices:

Bread or toast (whole grain), bagels, English muffins

Breadsticks

Cereal snack mix (prepare with margarine, garlic powder and Worcestershire sauce)

Cookies (homemade using whole grains, oils and minimal sugar)

Crackers

- No-fat commercial choices: Finn Crisps, Flatbread, Hardtack, Matzo, Wasa Brod, Akmak
- Low-fat commercial choices: Bread Sticks, Melba Toast, Rye Krisps, Zwieback, Graham Crackers
- Higher sodium choices: Oyster Crackers, Saltines, Soda Crackers

Dried fruits: apricots, dates, prunes, raisins

Frozen yogurt

Fruits and real fruit juices (fresh, frozen or canned in fruit juice)

Fruit and nut breads (prepared with whole grains, oils, and minimal sugar)

Fruit Roll-ups, Fruit Bars and Fruit Jerkey

Low-fat commercial snacks: animal crackers, gingersnaps, fig bars, graham crackers, molasses cookies

Nuts (unsalted and roasted)

Peanut butter

Peanuts (unsalted and roasted)

Popcorn (air-popped or popped in acceptable vegetable oils, served plain, lightly salted or sprinkled with parmesan cheese)

Pretzels (unsalted)

Sandwiches

Seeds (unsalted and roasted)

Soybeans (unsalted and roasted)

Trail mix (unsalted popcorn, raisins, unsalted peanuts, dates and dried fruits such as apricots, peaches, pears, and pineapple

Vegetables (raw, cooked or served with low-fat dips)

Eating Away From Home

It is possible to eat out and still watch your food choices. However, you need to pre-plan:

> **WHERE** you will eat.
> **WHAT** you will eat.
> **HOW MUCH** you will eat.

- ***Pre-plan where you will eat:*** Choose a restaurant that will help instead of hinder your self-management efforts. Pick a place with a varied menu where you will be able to find healthy alternatives.

- ***Pre-plan what you will eat:*** The following suggestions often work well.

For breakfast:

1. Choose cereals (hot or cold). Have them with low-fat or skim milk.
2. Try yogurt served over fruit.
3. If you choose eggs, limit yourself to one and have it poached or soft cooked.
4. Skip Danish, doughnuts or other pastries. Instead, try muffins (bran, corn, English); toast (whole wheat, rye, raisin); or bagels. Ask for them to be served "dry" and then add small amounts of margarine or butter.

For lunch:

1. Try salads with low-fat protein sources such as turkey, chicken, fish, yogurt or cottage cheese.
2. Sandwiches made with lean cuts of meat—turkey, chicken, ham, beef, etc.—are good choices. Avoid cold cuts and cheese. Ask for the mayonnaise on the side.
3. Salads—vegetable, cole slaw, bean salad—are good side dishes.

4. A plain grilled hamburger (quarter pound) will be a better choice than grilled cheese or frankfurter. It will also be a better choice than deep fat fried chicken and fish sandwiches.
5. Soups can also be excellent choices.
6. Fresh fruit, fruit cup, low-fat yogurt, fruit ices or sherbet are better dessert choices than cakes, pies or cookies.

For dinner:
1. Cocktails or liquor can add many calories. Have liquor mixed with water, juice, low-calorie soft drinks or club soda instead of pre-sweetened mixes. A glass of wine with club soda (a Spritzer) is a good choice. Sparkling water or juice is an even better choice. Avoid high-salt, high-fat snacks.
2. For an appetizer try melon or other fresh fruit or fruit juices, raw vegetables, broths, shellfish or low-calorie dip.
3. Ask for salad dressings on the side and use them sparingly. Mix your own oil and vinegar. Lemon juice and spices make an excellent low-calorie dressing.
4. Fish, poultry, lean meat or shellfish are good choices for an entree. Have them baked, broiled, poached, steamed, stir-fried or sauteed in small amounts of oil or margarine. Ask for a 4-ounce portion and have sauces or gravies served on the side. If you order beef, a filet mignon or shish kebob might be the best choices.
5. Choose a vegetable that is prepared without sauce or butter. Use lemon juice, vinegar and pepper as seasoning. Limit sour cream on potatoes. Instead, try unflavored yogurt or a little grated parmesan cheese, a dash of Worcestershire sauce and pepper, or lemon and pepper.
6. Be careful of dishes containing soy sauce and monosodium glutamate (MSG)—both are high in sodium. MSG can often be left out of a dish at your request.
7. The best choices for dessert are fresh fruit, fruit cup, fruit ice, or sherbet—or just taste a bit of someone else's.

At coffee break time:
1. Try fresh fruit, dried fruit, or juices.
2. Muffins, toast, English muffins or bagels are good choices.
3. Avoid pastries and doughnuts.

- ***Pre-plan how much you will eat.*** By planning how much you will eat, you can make adjustments in your exercise and food for the rest of the day. If you know the restaurant serves large portions, decide ahead of time that you will eat only part and bring the rest home to enjoy the following day.

If you do decide to have a dessert, consider sharing it with a friend or leaving some on the plate as restaurant critics do. One or two bites of very rich desserts usually provide 75 to 100 calories, 60 percent from fat.

RESTAURANT MENU CHOICES*
(One F stands for 5 grams of fat [one teaspoon] or 45 calories.)

Routine Choice	Pre-Planned Choice
BREAKFAST:	
Grapefruit half with sugar	Grapefruit half
2 fried eggs — FFF	Cereal with skim milk
Crisp bacon — FF	Canadian bacon — F
2 slices toast with butter and jelly — FFF	2 slices toast with margarine — FF
Whole milk — FF	Coffee black or with skim milk
2 cups coffee with cream and sugar — FF	
LUNCH:	
Cheeseburger on bun — FFFF	Chicken bouillon
French fries with ketchup — FFF	Sliced turkey sandwich on whole wheat bread — FF
Soft drink	Skim milk
DINNER:	
2 martinis	1 scotch and water
T-Bone, 12 oz. — FFFFFFFFFFFF	Filet, 7 oz. — FFFF
Baked potato with butter and sour cream — FFFF	Baked potato with 1 tsp. Margarine and pepper — F
Tossed salad w/French & blue cheese dressing — FFFFFFFFFF	Tossed salad w/oil and vinegar dressings — FFFF
Roll and butter — FF	Roll and margarine — F
Apple pie — FF	Fresh fruit cup
2 cups coffee w/cream and sugar — FF	Coffee, black or with skim milk

COMPARE:

	Routine Choice	Pre-Planned Choice
Total calories:	4,720	1,915
Calories as fat:	2,430	675
% calories as fat:	52%	34%

*Adapted from *Eater's Guide*, Candy Cummings and Vicky Newman.

- *Finally, practice assertiveness.* Firmly request that the food be prepared the way you want it. Assertiveness also means taking responsibility and initiative in social situations. For example, when you are eating out, order first. People generally follow the "trend" in social situations, and you can set the tone for the whole meal by your example. Remember, you are the customer. Fill out the suggestion cards and encourage restaurants to offer low fat, sugar and salt choices. Making small changes in selections away from home does pay off.

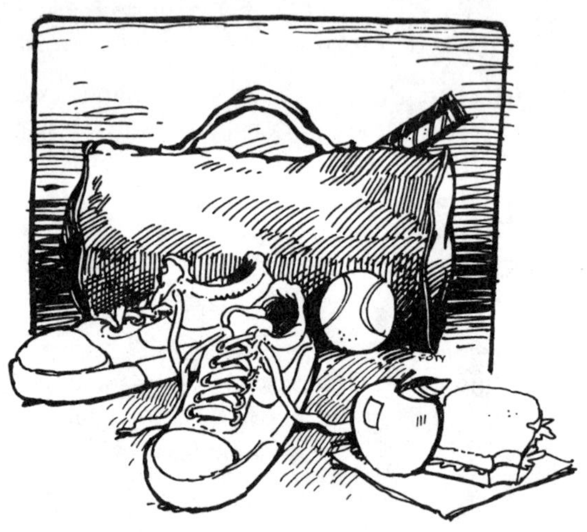

Nutrition for Athletes

Athletes, long considered the models of health and fitness, in general have eating habits so poor that they threaten their performance and endanger their health. This conclusion was reached following a four-year survey of 16 athletic teams at Syracuse University conducted by Sarah Short and published in 1983. The study showed wrestlers who literally starved themselves, eating as few as 78 calories a day, and football players who gorged themselves, wolfing down as many as 15,000 calories a day. Many of the athletes ate too much fat and salt, chewed tobacco, and drank too much. Others dehydrated themselves drastically to shed pounds quickly, their weights subsequently changing erratically and frequently. All of these are behaviors that can take a toll on an individual's health in the long run.

Fuel Metabolism During Exercise

Before we can make specific food recommendations we need to review how the body gets its fuel during exercise. There are three basic limiting factors to physical exertion: oxygen, water, and calories.

Deficits of these nutrients can occur singly or in combination. Under optimal conditions humans can survive about 10 minutes without oxygen, 18 days without water, and nearly 60 days without food. With exercise these times decrease drastically but stay in about the same proportions. Lack of oxygen (anaerobic activity) will stop the exerciser first; next, lack of water (dehydration); and finally, lack of food (glucose).

Carbohydrates and fat are the major fuel sources for exercise. During the first 20 to 30 minutes of exercise, the body utilizes glycogen, which is carbohydrate stored in the liver and muscles, as its primary fuel source. In endurance competition, carbohydrate initially furnishes 90 percent of the energy used and fat 10 percent. As competition increases, carbohydrate use decreases and the use of free fatty acids (from fat) increases. By the end of the competition, most of the energy used will be from fat. With improved fat utilization, depletion of glycogen is slowed and endurance enhanced. The ability to sustain prolonged vigorous exercise is directly related to the initial levels of muscle and liver glycogen. If you don't have glycogen you feel sluggish. When marathoners run out of glycogen they "hit the wall."

Exercise requires more carbohydrate but relatively no more protein than when a person is at rest. The average American eats two to three times as much protein as is required for body maintenance and growth and this will be very adequate for athletes as well. Excessive protein can deprive the athlete of more efficient fuel. Foods high in fat will contain more calories than will generally be needed. For the most part, body fat is an unnecessary burden.

Fluids and Exercise

When you exercise you can lose large amounts of water. This reduces the body's ability to provide adequate circulation to the working muscles and to your skin for dissipating heat. This can reduce athletic performance and even endanger health. In healthy individuals body water comprises 50 to 70 percent of the total body weight and 70 percent of the muscle. The higher the percentage of body fat, the lower the percentage of water, because fat contains less water than muscle.

The primary need of the sweating athlete is to replace the considerable amount of water lost. Thirst is not a good guide for how much to drink, because the thirst response in humans is blunted considerably during and immediately after vigorous exercise. Dehydration can also occur in cold or cool weather. When you exercise in cold weather, your body still sweats. To keep warm and yet allow sweat to evaporate, wear several layers of loose clothing. And remember, even in cold weather you still need to drink water.

Water is not the only component of sweat. Of the minerals lost in sweat, sodium and chloride (salt) are the most abundant. However, loss of sodium chloride is not what threatens an athlete during exercise. The kidneys and sweat glands can conserve sodium when it is in short supply. The kidneys control the body's water and mineral content. When the body is dehydrated, the kidneys cut back on urine production. They also conserve minerals so there is little danger of a shortage of sodium, potassium, or magnesium. A nutritious diet will supply all the sodium and potassium needed.

Since thirst is not a reliable indicator of water needs under pre-event stress and in warm environments, the athlete must plan ahead for optimum hydration. The hydrated state can be maintained by consuming fluid before, during and after exercise.

Water is absorbed into the system faster than juices and special electrolyte drinks that contain sugar, glucose, sodium, potassium and other ingredients. The more sugar or carbohydrate, the slower the rate of emptying. Sugar content of sports drinks should not exceed 2 to 2 1/2 grams per 100 milliliters (1/2 teaspoon of sugar in 1/2 cup water). Most commercial drinks have two to three times that amount of sugar. If used before, during or after exercise, they should be diluted by at least 50 percent—1/2 cup sport drink plus 1/2 cup water. In hot weather, cold water is absorbed faster. During the winter, skiers and hikers need to drink warm fluids, such as soup and cocoa, to prevent chilling the body core.

To avoid dehydration:

- Drink plenty of cool, plain water, before, during and after practice and competition as a preventive measure even if you don't feel thirsty.
- Two hours before an event drink 1 to 1 1/2 cups of plain, cool water.
- Ten to 15 minutes before an event drink 1 to 1 1/2 cups of plain, cool water.
- Every 10 to 15 minutes during the event drink 1/2 cup of water. After an event replace weight loss with fluids. For every pound lost as sweat replace it with 2 cups of water. Don't rely on thirst alone as to how much water your body needs.
- If water loss has been severe, the rehydration process may take 24 to 36 hours.
- Avoid sport drinks before or during exercise. They contain salt or sugar and are not absorbed by the body as quickly as water.
- Do not use salt tablets. Too much salt draws water into the stomach to dissolve and dilute it. Salt tablets can also irritate the stomach and cause nausea.

Nancy Clark's book, **The Athlete's Kitchen**, is a "how-to" book designed to improve daily training diets by giving tips on how to choose eat-on-the-run snacks, as well as sport-specific tips. Many of the suggestions in this section are adapted from her book.

Snacks Before Practice for Quick Energy

Avoid high sugar foods before practices. A large amount or high concentration of sweets—such as candy and pop—triggers the immediate release of high levels of insulin. With the extra insulin and exercise you may cause blood sugar to drop abnormally low. This may leave you feeling lightheaded, shaky, uncoordinated, and hungry. We already have all the "quick energy" we need stored in the liver in the form of glycogen.

To prevent low blood sugar (hypoglycemia), eat foods high in complex carbohydrate and low in fat, such as crackers, English muffins, bagels, bread sticks, muffins, yogurt, soups, etc., rather than sweets. Other carbohydrate foods such as bananas, apples, raisins and dried fruit contain "natural sugars" and also have vitamins and minerals so are good choices.

Meals the Night Before Competition

Eat a high carbohydrate meal the night before competition to increase glycogen stores. The following foods are suggested:

spaghetti	potatoes
muffins	milk
fruit juices	noodles
peas	dried fruits
pineapple	rice
crackers	dates
bananas	ice milk
rolls	

Avoid foods containing fat as well as carbohydrate, such as pizza and ice cream. To do this consider the following:

- Replace butter, margarine, or peanut butter with jam on toast, muffins, bagels.
- Replace donuts with English muffins, bagels.
- Replace cheese with low-fat crackers.
- Replace eggs with pancakes.
- Replace meat sauce on spaghetti with tomato sauce.
- Replace ice cream with ice milk or sherbet.

Meals the Day of Competition

On the day of competition eat a light breakfast and lunch. Toast, juice or fruit and cereal with skim milk are good breakfast choices. A turkey sandwich, skim milk and fruit are a good lunch.

A lighter pre-game meal three to four hours before the event allows the stomach to be empty at the time of competition. If exercise occurs immediately after ingesting food, gastrointestinal distress—nausea, vomiting, bloating, and cramping—can occur. Digestion of food and absorption of nutrients competes with muscle metabolism for blood supply, thus diminishing blood supply to working muscles.

A pre-game meal should contain some protein, a minimal amount of fat, and liberal amounts of complex carbohydrate. The menu can include lean meat (poultry without the skin, or fish), potatoes with no gravy, vegetables, bread with no butter, salad without dressing, fruit and skim milk.

Nutrients at Halftime or During Competition

During halftime or athletic events lasting several hours, watery fruits such as oranges are good choices. They provide a small amount of natural sugar to revive the athlete without overdosing on sugar. Other juicy fruits, such as apples, peaches, plums and pears are all "sugar boosts" as well as being 85 percent water.

Summary

The nutritional needs of most athletes can be met by a well balanced diet that satisfies the caloric demand of the sport. Food and nutrient supplements to a well-balanced diet are usually not needed. There is little evidence that such practices improve athletic performance. Athletic performance is affected by nutrition. So eat well and do your best!

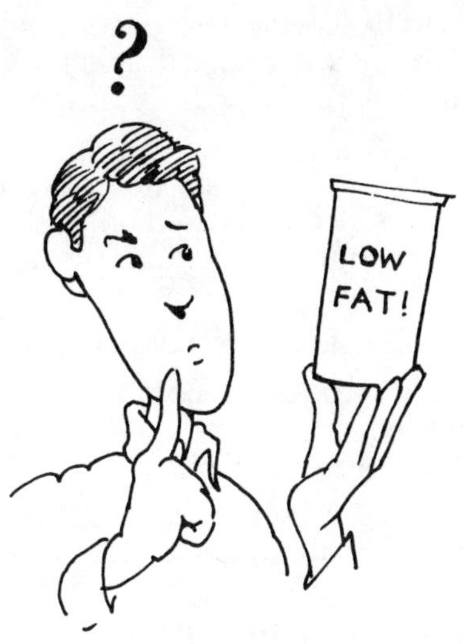

Being A Good Nutrition Consumer

Above all, be a good nutrition consumer. Frederick Stare, in his book **Eat O.K.—Feel O.K.**, points out that common sense is a hard product to sell. He wonders why it is so much easier for pseudo-scientists to sell food fads than it is for ethical scientists to convince people of the good nutrition that is easily obtainable in our ordinary foods.

Food and medical faddism and quackery are harmful. If you are taken in by misinformation, you stand a very good chance of endangering your own health as well as that of your family. Putting your faith in the curative powers of some "magic" food or formula can lead to neglect of a real disorder.

The fantastic drain on the family pocketbook is one of the greatest hazards of food quackery. Vitamin and mineral preparations, gimmicks, reducing pills, misleading books, diet plans, "organic" foods, and fancy machines and devices cost the American public an enormous sum of money each year. Fads also raise false hopes in those who think their aches and pains may disappear if they take the nutritional supplements or advice.

How can you spot the quack or faddist who spreads misinformation for personal profit? Look for the following characteristics:*

1. They always have something to sell: a course of lectures, pills, nature foods, tonics, food supplements, diet plans, rollers (to roll off fat), books, even pots and pans.
2. They guarantee quick cures—on a money-back basis—"if your arthritis isn't cured in eight days."

3. They often claim to be "medical experts" or "nutritionists" with some secret formula or knowledge that will cure, and they usually boast about membership in a "scientific society" with a high-sounding name.
4. They use testimonials and case histories to prove that their product is miraculous, not facts based on carefully controlled studies published in reputable medical journals and confirmed by independent researchers.
5. They distort scientific data to suit their own ends.
6. They say that what you are doing now is deadly—the food you are eating is poisoned, the way you cook it is all wrong.
7. They claim to be persecuted by the medical establishment or governmental agencies, insisting that the medical profession and the Food and Drug Administration are corrupt and influenced by big business.

*From: **Eat OK — Feel OK!** Fredrick J. Stare, M.D., Elizabeth M. Whelan, Sc.D.

Remember, the faddist and quack isn't interested in you—just your bank account. Be a wise consumer. Make eating choices that work and that you enjoy.

WHERE TO READ ABOUT NUTRITION

General Nutrition:

Jane Brody's Nutrition Book
Jane Brody
W.W. Norton and Co.
New York, London 1981

Eat O.K.—Feel O.K.
Fredrick Stare and Elizabeth Whelan
Christopher Publishing House
North Quincy, MA 1978

Your Basic Guide to Nutrition
Fredrick Stare and Virginia Aronson
George F. Stickley Co.
Philadelphia, PA 1984

Reader's Digest Eat Better, Live Better: A Common Sense Guide to Nutrition and Good Health
The Reader's Digest Association
Random House
New York, NY 1982

Eater's Guide—Nutrition Basics for Busy People
Candy Cumming and Vicky Newman
Prentice-Hall, Inc.
Englewood Cliffs, NJ 1981

Vitamins & "Health" Foods: The Great American Hustle
Victor Herbert and Stephen Barrett
George F. Stickley Co.
Philadelphia, PA 1981

A Guide to Healthy Eating: What You Need to Know About Fat, Cholesterol, Fiber and Salt**
Marion Franz, Betsy Kerr Hedding, Karen Holtmeier, Arlene Monk, and Dorothy Siemers
Park Nicollet Medical Foundation
Minneapolis, MN 1982, 1985

Weight Loss:

Shapedown Weight Management Program for Adolescents
Laurel Mellin
Balboa Publishing
San Francisco, CA 1983

The Weight Watcher's 365 Day Menu Cookbook
Weight Watcher's International
New American Library Books
New York, NY 1983

Thinward Bound Medical Management of Weight Loss**
Mary Jane Madden and Donna Hoel
Robert J. Brady Co.
Bowie, MD 1983

California Diet and Exercise Program
Peter Wood
Anderson World Books
Mountain View, CA 1983

Vegetarian:

Diet for a Small Planet: Tenth Anniversary Edition
Frances Moore Lappe
Ballantine Books
Westminster, MD 1982

Eating for the Eighties: A Complete Guide to Vegetarian Nutrition
Joan Coulter Hartbarger and Neil J. Hartbarger
Saunders Press
Philadelphia, PA 1981

Laurel's Kitchen, A Handbook for Vegetarian Cookery and Nutrition
Robertson, Flinders and Godfrey
Nilgiri Press
Petaluma, CA
Bantam Books
New York, NY 1976

Moosewood Cookbook
Mollie Katzen
Ten Speed Press
Berkeley, CA 1977

Fitness:

The Athlete's Kitchen
Nancy Clark
Bantam Books
New York, NY 1983

The Nautilus Nutrition Book
Ellington Darden
Contemporary Books 1981

Fit or Fat
Covert Bailey
Houghton Mifflin Co.
Boston, MA 1978

Children:

Feeding Your Baby With Love
Irene Alton and Norman Vernig
Twin Cities Dietetic Association
St. Paul, MN 1981

Child of Mine: Feeding With Love and Good Sense
Ellyn Satter
Bull Publishing Co.
Palo Alto, CA 1983

Pregnancy:

Nutrition for Your Pregnancy—The University of Minnesota Guide
Judith E. Brown
University of Minnesota Press
Minneapolis, MN 1983

Pickles and Ice Cream, The Complete Guide to Nutrition During Pregnancy
Mary Abbott Hess and Anne Elise Hunt
McGraw-Hill Book Co.
New York, NY 1982

Gestational Diabetes: Guidelines for a Safe Pregnancy and Healthy Baby**
Marion Franz, Nancy Cooper and Lucy Mullen
International Diabetes Center
Minneapolis, MN 1985

More Than "Just Cookbooks":

Craig Claiborne's Gourmet Diet
Craig Claiborne
Time Books, Alexandria VA 1980
Ballantine Books, Westminster, MD 1981
Harper & Row, New York, NY 1980

You've Got It Made: Make Ahead Meals for Your Family and for Cooperative Dinner Parties
Marian Burros
William Morrow and Company
New York, NY 1985

AHA Minnesota Grocery Guide
American Heart Association
Minnesota Affiliate, Inc.
Minneapolis, MN 1982

Cooking to Stay in SHAPE**
Marion Franz and Betsy Kerr Hedding
SHAPE, Park Nicollet Medical Center
Minneapolis, MN 1983

Cooking Without Your Salt Shaker
American Heart Association
Minnesota Affiliate, Inc.
Minneapolis, MN 1978

Lean Cuisine: Delicious Recipes for the Healthy Stay Slender Life
Barbara Gibbons and the Editors of Consumer Guide
Harper and Row
New York, NY 1979

The American Heart Association Cookbook
David McKay Co.
New York, NY 1984
Ballantine Books
New York, NY 1979

Family Cookbook II
The American Diabetes Association and American Dietetic Association
Prentice-Hall
Englewood Cliffs, NJ 1983

Microwave Cooking on a Diet
Litton Microwave Cooking Products
Publication Arts, Inc.
Minnetonka, MN 1980

Special Concerns:

Exchanges for All Occasions—Meeting the Challenge of Diabetes**
(Variations of the Exchange System of Meal Planning to Help People with Diabetes Enjoy Holidays, Ethnic Foods, Dining Out and Other Occasions)
Marion Franz
International Diabetes Center
Minneapolis, MN 1983

Convenience Food Facts**
(Nutrient Content—Calories, Carbohydrate, Protein, Fat, and Sodium—Plus Exchange Values for more than 1500 Popular Name-Brand Processed Foods)
Arlene Monk and Marion Franz
International Diabetes Center
Minneapolis, MN 1984, 1985

Fast Food Facts**
(Nutrient Content and Exchange Values for Menu Items from 21 Popular Fast-Food Restaurant Chains)
Marion Franz
International Diabetes Center
Minneapolis, MN 1983, 1985

Adding Fiber to Your Diet**
Nutrition Section of the Health Education Dept., and International Diabetes Center
Park Nicollet Medical Foundation
Minneapolis, MN 1984

**Books Available at the Park Nicollet Medical Foundation and International Diabetes Center, 5000 West 39th Street, Minneapolis, MN 55416.

BIBLIOGRAPHY

Chapter 1

American Cancer Society. Conference on Nutrition in Cancer Causation and Prevention. **Cancer Research** 43(5), 1983.

American Council on Science and Health: **The Effects of Caffeine** Summit, NJ, 1983.

American Diabetes Association. Special Report: Principles of nutrition and dietary recommendations for individuals with diabetes mellitus, 1979. **Diabetes** 28(11):1027-1030, 1979.

American Heart Association: **Eating for a Healthy Heart. Dietary Treatment of Hyperlipidemia** New York City, 1983.

American Heart Association Committee on Nutrition: **Diet and Coronary Heart Disease** New York City, 1965, revised 1968, 1973, 1978.

Anderson J, Chen WL, Sieling B: **Plant Fiber Source Book** Lexington, KY, HCF Diabetes Research Foundation, Inc, 1980.

Arky R, Wylie-Rosett J, El-Beheri B: Examination of current dietary recommendations for individuals with diabetes mellitus. **Diabetes Care** 5:59-63, 1982.

Breslow L: Prospects for improving health through reducing risk factors. **Preventive Medicine** 7:449-458, 1978.

Brewster L, Jacobson MF: **The Changing American Diet** Washington, DC, Center for Science in the Public Interest, 1982.

Bunker ML, McWilliams M: Caffeine content of common beverages. **Journal of the American Dietetic Association** 74:28, 1979.

Carroll K: Breast cancer and total fat intake. **Progress in Biochemistry and Pharmacology** Vol 10, 1975.

Curatolo P, Robertson D: The health consequences of caffeine. **Annals of Internal Medicine** 98:641, 1983.

Dahl JK: Salt and hypertension. **American Journal of Clinical Nutrition** 25:231-244, 1972.

Dietary Guidelines Advisory Committee Report: Nutrition and your health; dietary guidelines for Americans. **Nutrition Today** 20:8-15, 1985.

Enos WF, Holmes RH, Beyer JC: Coronary disease among United States soldiers killed in action in Korea. **Journal of the American Medical Association** 152:1090-1093, 1953.

Enos WF, Beyer JC, Holmes RH: Pathogenesis of coronary disease in American soldiers killed in Korea. **Journal of the American Medical Association** 158:912-914, 1955.

Gotto AM, Bierman EL, Connor WE, et al: AHA Special Report. Recommendations for treatment of hyperlipidemia in adults. **Circulation** 69:1065A-1090A, 1984.

Heaney RP: The role of diet and activity in the treatment of osteoporosis. In: **Diet and Exercise: Synergism in Health Maintenance.** Editors: White PL, Mondeika T; Chicago, American Medical Association, 1982.

The Joint National Committee on Detection, Education, and Treatment of High Blood Pressure: The 1984 report. **Archives of Internal Medicine** 144:1045-1057, 1984.

The Lipid Research Clinics Program: The Lipid Research Clinics coronary primary prevention trial results. I. Reduction in incidence of coronary heart disease. II. The relationship of reduction in incidence of coronary heart disease to cholesterol lowering. **Journal of the American Medical Association** 251(3):351-363, 365-373, 1984.

Marston RM, Welsh SO: Nutrient content of the U.S. food supply, 1982. **National Food Review** 25:7, 1984.

National Center for Health Statistics: **Health and Nutrition Examination Survey (HANES), Advance Data** No. 54, February 1981.

National Center for Health Statistics: **Monthly Vital Statistics Report** 29: No. 13, 1981.

National Institutes of Health: Consensus Development Conference statement: **Lowering Blood Cholesterol to Prevent Heart Disease** Vol. 5, Number 7, 1984.

National Research Council Committee on Diet, Nutrition, and Cancer: **Diet, Nutrition, Cancer** Washington, DC, 1982.

Notelovitz M, Wane M: **The Informed Woman's Guide to Preventing Osteoporosis.** Triad Publishing Co, Inc, Gainesville, FL, 1982.

Osteoporosis. **Consumer Reports** pp. 576-580, October 1984.

Packard V: **Processed Foods and the Consumer.** Minneapolis, University of Minnesota Press, 1976.

Palmer S: Diet, nutrition and cancer: the future of dietary policy. **Cancer Research (Supplement)** 43:2509S-2514S, 1983.

Palmer S, Bakshi K: Diet, nutrition, and cancer: interim dietary guidelines. **Journal of National Cancer Institute** 70(6):1153-1170, 1983.

Rationale of the diet-heart statement of the American Heart Association. **Circulation** 65:839A, 1982.

Turpeineu O: Effect of cholesterol-lowering diet on mortality from coronary heart disease and other causes. **Circulation** 59:1, 1979.

US Department of Agriculture: The sodium content of your food. **Home and Garden Bulletin No.233** Washington, DC, 1980.

US Department of Agriculture and US Department of Health, Education and Welfare: **Nutrition and Your Health; Dietary Guidelines for Americans** Washington, DC, US Government Printing Office, February 1980.

US Senate Select Committee on Nutrition and Human Needs: **Dietary Goals for the United States, 2nd edition** Washington, DC, US Government Printing Office, December 1977.

Van Itallie TB: Obesity: adverse effects on health and longevity. **American Journal of Clinical Nutrition** 32:2723-2733, 1979.

West KM, Kalbfleisch JM: Influence of nutritional factors on prevalence of diabetes. **Diabetes** 20:99-108, 1971.

Chapter 2

Clark N: **The Athlete's Kitchen** Boston, CBI Publishing Co, Inc, 1981.

Hockey R: Body frame size, determination by wrist measurement. In **Physical Fitness** St. Louis, Mosby, 1977.

Zuti B, Golding A: Comparing diet and exercise as weight reduction tools. **Physician and Sportsmedicine** June 1976.

Chapters 3, 4 and 5

Anderson J, Chen WL, Sieling B: **Plant Fiber Source Book** Lexington, KY, HCF Diabetes Research Foundation, Inc, 1980.

The Buying Guide for Fresh Fruits, Vegetables, Herbs and Nuts Hagerstown, MD, Blue Goose, Inc, 1980.

Franz M: Is aspartame safe? **The Diabetes Educator** 10:56-57, 1984.

Monk A, Franz M: **Convenience Food Facts** Minneapolis, International Diabetes Center, 1984, revised 1985.

Multiple Risk Factor Intervention Trial (MRFIT) Research Group: **Progressive Eating Guide** Minneapolis, 1979.

National Livestock and Meat Board: **Nutritive Value of Meat** Chicago, 1976

New York Heart Association Diet Committee: **The Culinary Hearts Kitchen Course** New York City, 1982

Oregon Heart Association: **Discovering Low-Fat Cheeses** Portland, OR, 1978

Pennington JAT, Church HN: **Bowes and Church Food Values of Portions Commonly Used** 13th Edition, Harper & Row, 1980.

US Dept. of Agriculture Nutrient Composition Laboratory, Nutrition Institute, Human Nutrition Center, Beltsville, MD, **Journal of Food Science** 45:130-144, 1980; 46:425-427, 1981.

US Dept. of Agriculture: The sodium content of your food. **Home and Garden Bulletin No. 233** Washington, DC, US Government Printing Office, 1980.

US Dept. of Agriculture: **Nutritive Value of American Foods** Agriculture Handbook No. 456, Washington, DC, US Government Printing Office, 1976.

US Dept. of Health and Human Services: **A Word About Low-Sodium Diets** HHS Publication 84-2179, Rockville, MD, 1984.

Vermeulen RT, Sedor FA, Kimm SYS: Effect of water rinsing on sodium content of selected foods. **Journal of the American Dietetic Association** 82:394-396, 1983.

Chapters 6, 7, 8, and 9

American Council on Science and Health: **The Health Effects of Caffeine** Summit, NJ, January, 1983.

Brody J: **Jane Brody's Nutrition Book** New York City, W.W. Norton Co., 1981.

Bunker ML, McWilliams M: Caffeine content of common beverages. **Journal of the American Dietetic Association** 74:28, 1979.

Curatolo P, Robertson D: The health consequences of caffeine. **Annals of Internal Medicine** 98:641, 1983.

Institute of Food Technology: Caffeine, a scientific status summary by IFT's expert panel on food safety and nutrition. **Food Technology** 37:87, April 1983

Institute of Nutrition: **Caffeine** Chapel Hill, NC, University of North Carolina, May 1981.

Chapter 10

AHA Minnesota Grocery Guide Minneapolis, American Heart Association Minnesota Affiliate, Inc, 1982.

Brody J: **Jane Brody's Nutrition Book** New York City, W.W. Norton Co, 1981.

Clark N: **The Athlete's Kitchen** Boston, CBI Publishing Co, 1981.

Cummings C, Newman U: **Eater's Guide** Englewood Cliffs, NJ, Prentice-Hall, Inc, 1981.

Short SA, Short W: Four-year study of university athlete's dietary intake. **Journal of the American Dietetic Association** 82:632, 1983.

Stare F, Whelan E: **Eat O.K.—Feel O.K.** North Quincy, MA, Christopher Publishing House, 1978.

INDEX